Table Of Contents

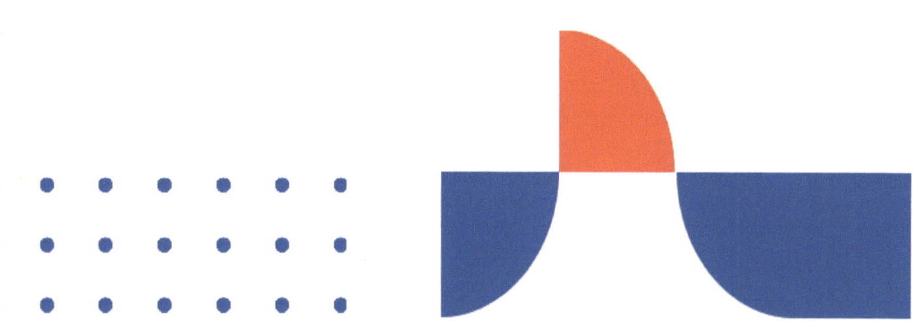

Chapter 1: Understanding Type 2 Diabetes

What is Type 2 Diabetes ?

History

Diabetes mellitus (DM) has been recognized for thousands of years. Greek word diabetes meaning "passing too much urine." Latin word mellitus meaning "sweet". Hence Diabetes means "Passing excessive sweet urine". Ancient Hindu writings discussed the disease of madhumeha, which means "honey urine."

Diabetes is a group of metabolic diseases characterized by-

Hyperglycemia (increased blood sugar)- that occurs either when the pancreas does not produce enough insulin or when the body cannot effectively use the insulin it produces.

Diabetes in India

India is now the diabetes capital of world. According to WHO report in India, there are estimated **77 million** people above the age of 18 years are suffering from **diabetes (type 2)** and nearly **25 million** are **prediabetics** (at a higher risk of developing diabetes in near future).

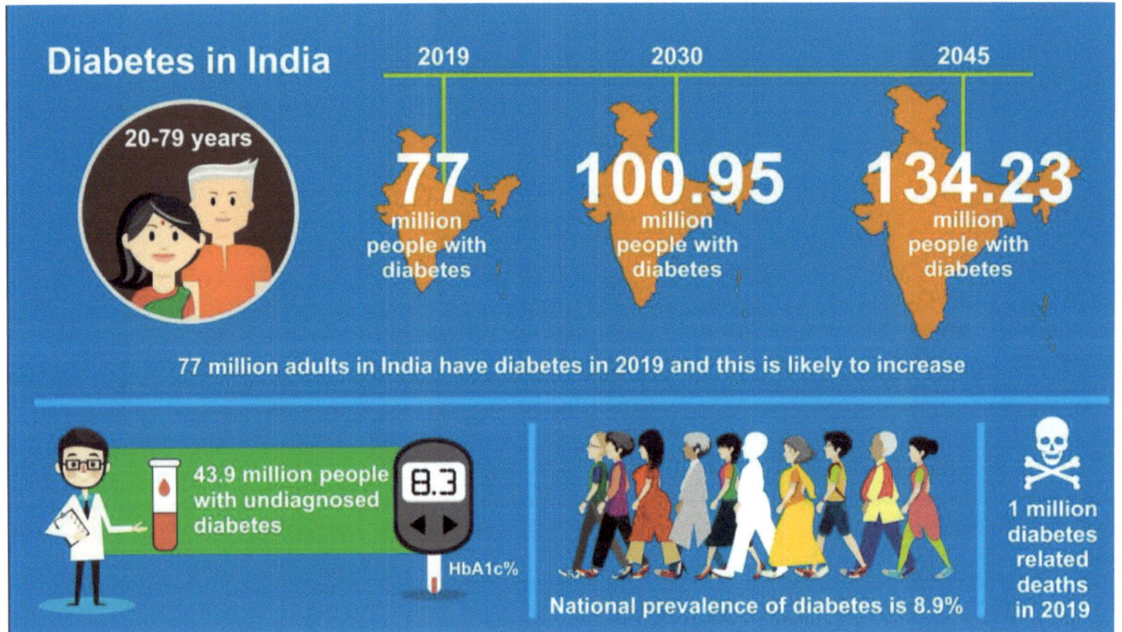

Causes and Risk Factors

One of the primary causes of type 2 diabetes is **insulin resistance**. Insulin is a hormone that helps regulate blood sugar levels by allowing glucose to enter cells for energy production. When the body becomes resistant to insulin, glucose builds up in the bloodstream, leading to high blood sugar levels. This can eventually result in the development of type 2 diabetes.

While genetics play a role in predisposing individuals to diabetes, lifestyle factors such as **diet** and **exercise** also play a crucial role in determining whether or not someone will develop the disease. By making positive lifestyle changes, individuals can reduce their risk of developing type 2 diabetes, even if they have a genetic predisposition.

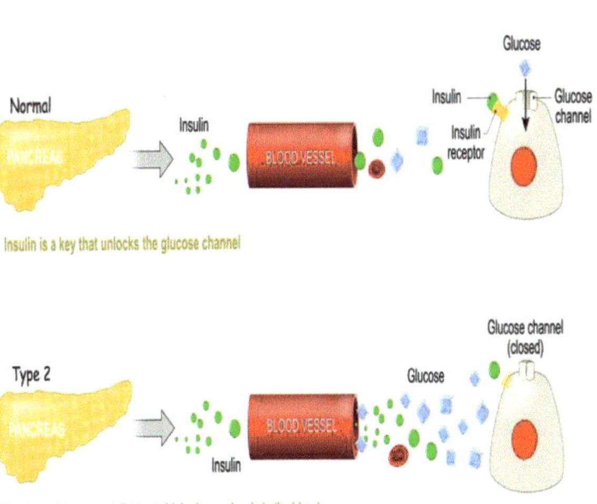

CAUSES OF TYPE 2 DIABETES

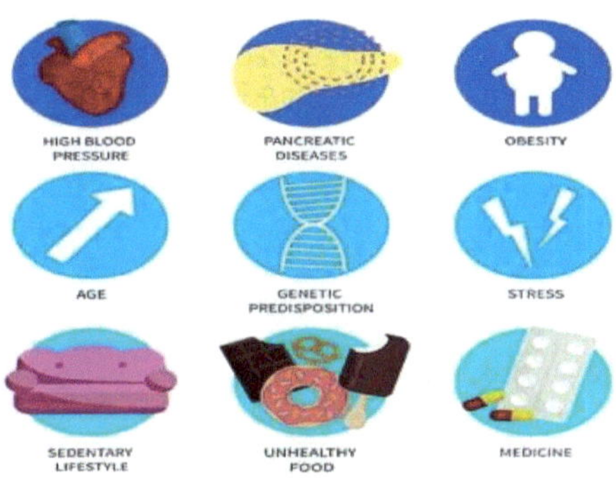

Factors such as **obesity, physical inactivity**, and **poor diet** can contribute to insulin resistance and increase the risk of developing diabetes.

Another significant risk factor for type 2 diabetes is **genetics**. Individuals with a family history of diabetes are at a higher risk of developing the condition themselves.

Additionally, **age** and **ethnicity** can also influence the risk of developing type 2diabetes.
As individuals age, their risk of developing diabetes increases, particularly after the age of 45. Certain ethnic groups, such as African Americans, Hispanic Americans, and Native Americans, are also at a higher risk of developing diabetes compared to other populations. Understanding these risk factors can help individuals take proactive steps to prevent or manage the condition.

Other risk factors for type 2 diabetes include **high blood pressure, abnormal cholesterol levels**, and a **history of gestational diabetes**. Individuals with these risk factors should be especially vigilant about monitoring their blood sugar levels and making lifestyle changes to reduce their risk of developing diabetes.

Symptoms and Diagnosis

Symptoms of Type 2 diabetes can vary from person to person, but some common signs to watch out for include

- increased thirst
- frequent urination,
- rapid, unexplained weight loss,
- increased hunger despite weight loss,
- fatigue.
- numbness over hands & feet etc.

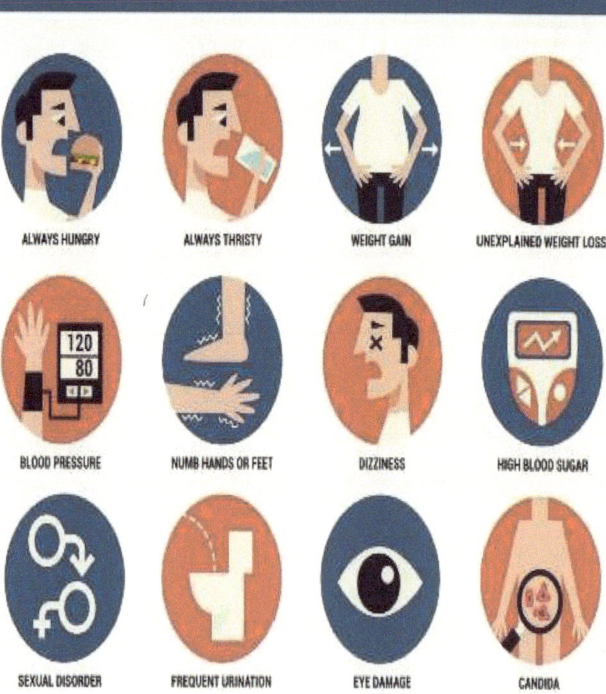

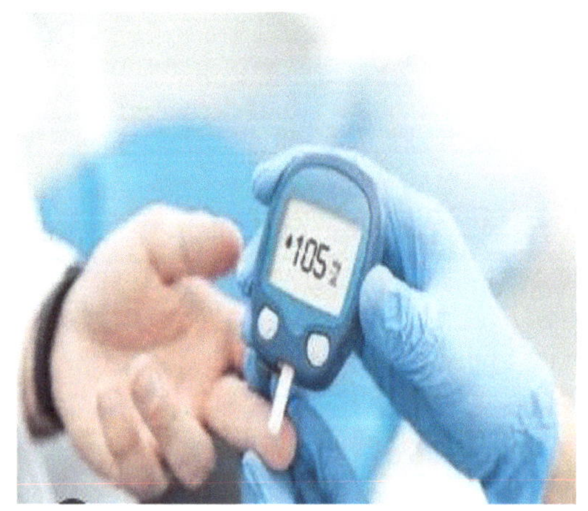

Diagnosing Type 2 diabetes typically involves a series of tests, including a fasting blood sugar test, oral glucose tolerance test, and A1C test. Diagnostic criteria for Diabetes:

- **Fasting blood glucose > 126 mg/dL**

  OR

- **2hour blood glucose >200 mg/dL**

  OR

- **A1C>6.5%**

Insulin Resistance & Diabetes Reversal

Type 2 diabetes is due to insulin resistance and it remains untreated if only medications are given. The root cause of the hyperglycemia in type 2 diabetes is high insulin resistance. Until we treat the root cause, insulin resistance , type 2 diabetes and all its complications will continue to get worse. **Insulin resistance** emerges, on average, almost **thirteen years** prior to **type 2 diabetes**

Diabetes Remission: is defined as a return of HbA1c to<6.5% that occurs spontaneously
or following an intervention and persists for atleast three months without usual glucose lowering pharmacotherapy.

Diabetes Reversal: means achieving normal blood sugar levels over an extended period without medication by life style modification.

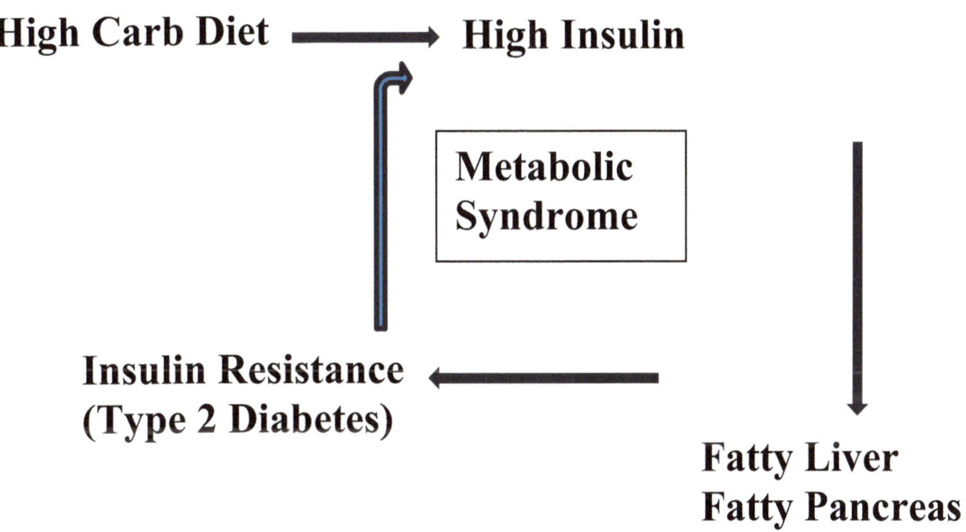

Chapter 2:
Conventional Treatments for Type 2 Diabetes

Medications for Diabetes Management

Diabetes medications and insulin are commonly prescribed to help control blood sugar levels and prevent complications associated with diabetes. These treatments work by either **increasing insulin production, improving insulin sensitivity, reducing glucose production in the liver, slowing down carbohydrate absorption in the intestines, increasing glucose excretion in the urine.** They can be effective in lowering blood sugar levels and managing symptoms, but they're not without their limitations. Let's take a closer look at the different types of medications and insulin therapy used in diabetes management. Some common types of oral medications include **metformin, sulfonylureas, thiazolidinediones, and DPP-4 inhibitors**. While these medications can be effective in lowering blood sugar levels, they may also have side effects such as gastrointestinal upset, weight gain, and hypoglycemia.

However **Acarbose, SGLT2 inhibitors, and GLP-1 analogs** all lower glucose but also lower insulin and cause weight loss. Since type 2 diabetes is a disease characterized by elevations in both blood glucose and blood insulin, these medications would be predicted to have the best outcome.

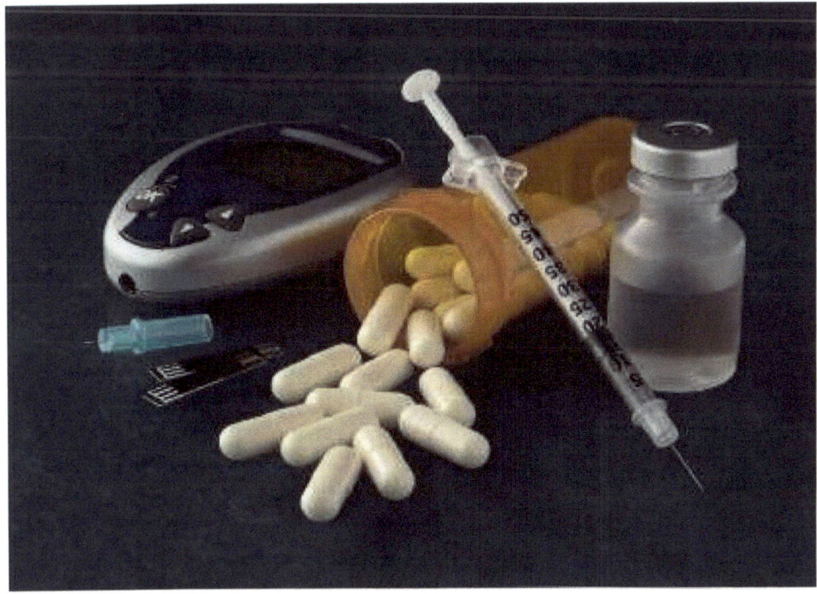

Insulin Therapy

 In addition to oral medications, insulin therapy is often prescribed for individuals with type 1 diabetes and some people with type 2 diabetes who require additional insulin support. Insulin can be administered through injections or insulin pumps and is essential for regulating blood sugar levels and preventing complications of diabetes. While insulin therapy is highly effective in controlling blood sugar levels, it can be challenging to manage and may require frequent adjustments to dosage and timing. Some individuals may also experience side effects such as **weight gain, hypoglycemia, and injection site reactions**.

Despite their effectiveness, conventional diabetes treatments have limitations that need to be considered. For example, medications and insulin therapy primarily focus on managing symptoms rather than addressing the underlying causes of diabetes. They may also come with risks and side effects that can impact quality of life. Additionally, these treatments do not necessarily reverse the progression of diabetes or prevent long-term complications associated with the condition. As such, individuals with diabetes may benefit from exploring complementary and alternative therapies that focus on addressing the root causes of the disease and promoting overall health and well-being.

In conclusion, while conventional treatments such as medications and insulin therapy play a crucial role in diabetes management, it's important to recognize their limitations and potential drawbacks. Some diabetes drugs are more likely to cause hypoglycemia, especially insulin and sulfonylureas. **Metformin, DPP-4 inhibitors, and SGLT2 inhibitors** have a lower risk of hypoglycemia, so these are preferred.

Chapter 3:
The Role of Nutrition in Diabetes Reversal

Nutrition is not just about counting calories; it's about fueling your body with the right nutrients to support overall health and well-being. Nutrition is the cornerstone of diabetes management, influencing blood sugar levels, insulin sensitivity, and overall health. By making informed dietary choices individuals with diabetes can optimize their blood sugar control and improve their quality of life. But what does a diabetes-friendly diet look like? Let's break it down.

LOW CARB HEALTHY FAT DIET(LCHF)

At its core, a diabetes-friendly **LCHF diet** emphasizes whole, unprocessed foods that are rich in nutrients and low in refined sugars and unhealthy fats. This includes plenty of fruits, vegetables, whole grains, lean proteins, and healthy fats. These foods provide essential vitamins, minerals, fiber and antioxidants that support overall health and help regulate blood sugar levels. One key principle of a diabetes-friendly diet is carbohydrate management. Carbohydrates are the primary macronutrient that affects blood sugar levels, so it's essential to choose carbohydrates wisely and monitor portion sizes. Focus on **complex carbohydrates** such as whole grains, legumes, fruits, and vegetables, which are rich in fiber and digest more slowly, leading to more stable blood sugar levels. Limit simple carbohydrates such as refined sugars and processed foods, which can cause rapid spikes in blood sugar.

In addition to managing carbohydrates, it's important to pay attention to the quality and quantity of protein and fat in your diet. Including **lean proteins** such as poultry, fish, tofu, and legumes can help promote satiety and stabilize blood sugar levels. **Healthy fats** from sources such as avocados, nuts, seeds, and olive oil can also support heart health and improve insulin sensitivity.

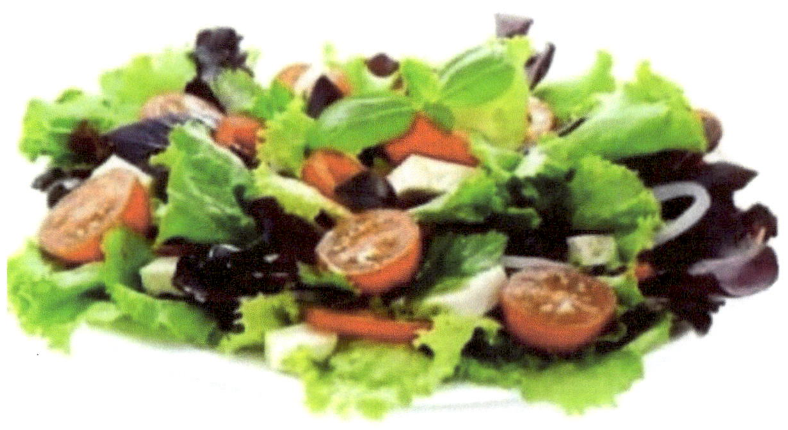

MEAL TIMING &
INTERMITTENT FASTING

Another important aspect of nutrition for diabetes management is **meal timing and distribution**. Eating regular, balanced meals and snacks throughout the day can help prevent large fluctuations in blood sugar levels and promote better overall control.

Intermittent fasting prevents the development of insulin resistance by creating extended periods of low insulin that maintain the body's sensitivity to insulin. This is the key to reversing prediabetes and type 2 diabetes.

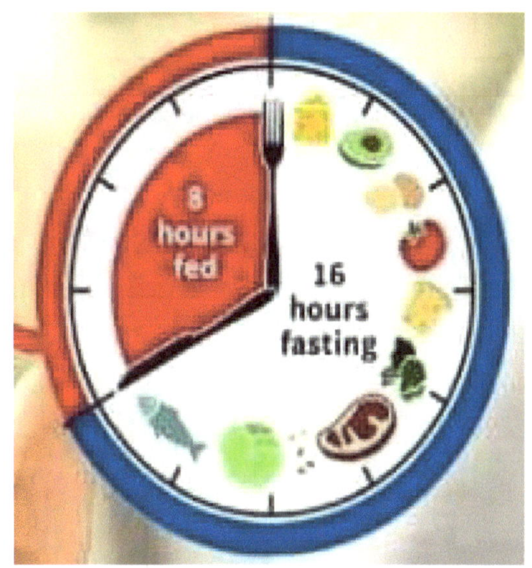

Intermittent fasting is an eating pattern that cycles between periods of eating and fasting. Intermittent fasting prevents the development of insulin resistance by creating extended periods of low insulin that maintain the body's sensitivity to insulin. This is the key to reversing prediabetes and type 2 diabetes. During fasting, glycogen stored in the liver is burnt first then body fat is used. Basal metabolism stays high, and instead of using food as fuel, stored body fat is used.

Types of Intermittent Fasting:

1. 5:2 Fasting
The idea is to eat normally for five days (don't count calories); then on the other two days, eat 500 or 600 calories a day, for women and men, respectively.

The 5:2 Method	DAY 1	DAY 2	DAY 3	DAY 4	DAY 5	DAY 6	DAY 7
	Eat normaly	FAST (500 to 600 kcal)	Eat normally	Eat normally	FAST(500 – 600 kcal)	Eat normaly	Eat normaly

2. Time-Restricted Fasting
With this type of intermittent fasting, you choose an eating window every day. For example on 16:8 plan, you consume food 8 hours a day, fasting for the other 16 hours.

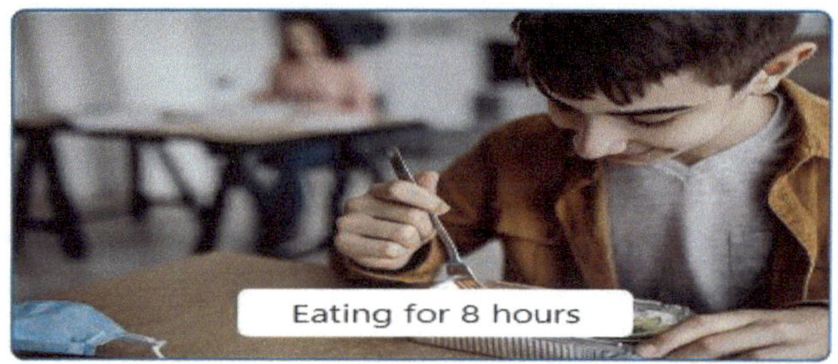

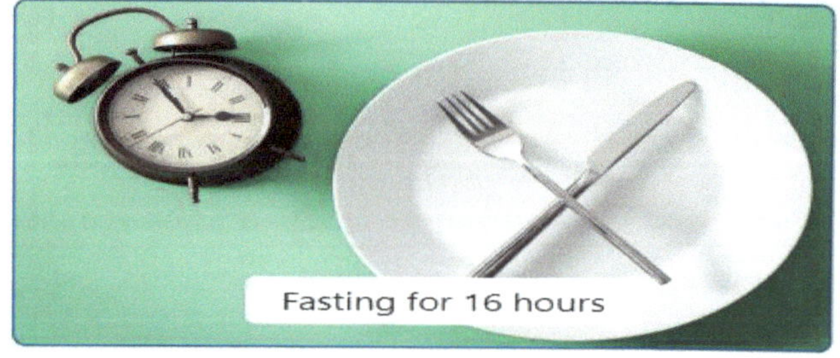

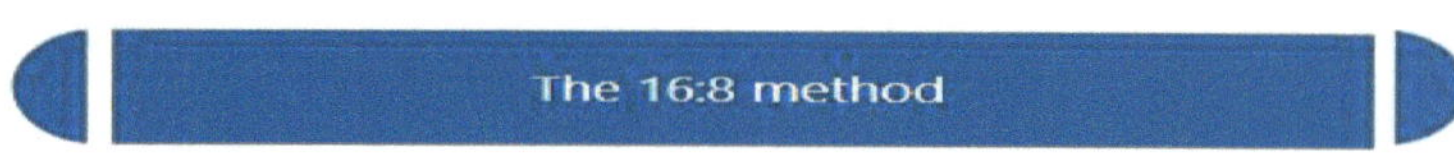

3.Alternate-Day Fasting
People might fast every other day, with a "fast" consisting of 25 percent of their calorie needs (about 500 calories), and non fasting days being normal eating days. This is a popular approach for weight loss. In fact, research found that, in overweight adults, alternate-day fasting significantly reduced body mass index, weight, fat mass, and total cholesterol.

"Fasting promotes autophagy, the natural 'cellular housekeeping' process where the body clears debris and other things that stand in the way of the health of mitochondria, which begins when liver glycogen is depleted,"

MEAL PORTIONS, MINDFUL EATING & HYDRATION

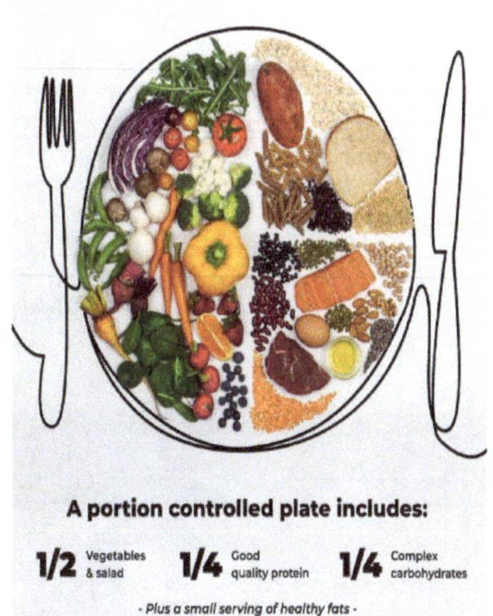

MEAL PORTIONS:

Meal portions for diabetic and obese patients are crucial for managing blood sugar levels and promoting weight loss.

Here are some general guidelines:

Encourage filling half the plate with non-starchy vegetables like leafy greens, broccoli, peppers, and tomatoes. A quarter of the plate can be lean protein such as chicken, fish, tofu, or beans, and the remaining quarter with whole grains or starchy vegetables like brown rice, quinoa, sweet potatoes, or whole grain pasta. Focus on healthy fats like those found in avocados, nuts, seeds, and olive oil. Limit saturated and trans fats found in fried foods, fatty cuts of meat, and processed snack. High- fiber foods like fruits, vegetables, whole grains, and legumes can help regulate blood sugar levels and promote feelings of fullness.

MINDFUL EATING:

Mindful eating practices such as paying attention to hunger and fullness cues, savoring each bite, and eating slowly can help prevent overeating and promote better digestion and nutrient absorption. Practice mindful eating at each meal to foster a healthier relationship with food and support your diabetes management goals. ☐

HYDRATION:

Adequate hydration is essential for overall health and can also help control appetite. Encourage drinking water throughout the day and limit sugary beverages

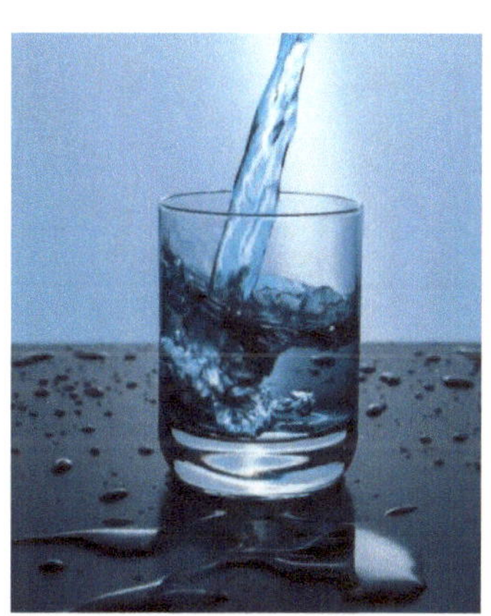

In conclusion, nutrition plays a crucial role in diabetes management and can even help reverse the condition. By focusing on LCHF diet, Meal timing. portion and practicing mindful eating, individuals with diabetes can optimize their blood sugar control and improve their overall health and wellbeing.

Chapter 4:
Exercise Strategies for Diabetes Management

Importance of Exercise in Diabetes Reversal

Exercise isn't just about burning calories or sculpting your physique—it's a powerful tool for **improving insulin sensitivity, lowering blood sugar levels, and boosting overall health and well-being.** One of the key benefits of exercise for individuals with type 2 diabetes is its ability to help control weight. **Maintaining a healthy weight** is crucial for managing diabetes as excess weight can lead to insulin resistance and higher blood sugar levels. By incorporating regular physical activity into your routine, you can help shed excess pounds and improve your overall health. Aim for at least **150 minutes** of moderate-intensity exercise per week, spread out over several days. In addition to weight management, exercise can also help **reduce stress levels** and improve mental health. Living with diabetes can be stressful, and exercise can be a great way to relieve tension and improve your mood. Physical activity releases **endorphins**, which are natural mood boosters, and can help alleviate symptoms of anxiety and depression. Incorporating exercise into your routine can have a positive impact on both your physical and mental well-being. Exercise comes in all shapes and sizes, and the key is finding activities that you enjoy and that fit seamlessly into your lifestyle. Whether you're a fan of high-intensity interval training **(HIIT)**, yoga, cycling, dancing, or simply taking a brisk walk around the neighborhood, there's a workout for everyone! ⬜. Exercise isn't just about what you do in the gym—it's also about how you move throughout your day. We'll discuss the importance of **NEAT** (non-exercise activity thermogenesis) and ways to increase your daily movement, from taking the stairs instead of the elevator to parking farther away from your destination and incorporating more activity breaks into your workday. Every little bit adds up, so don't underestimate the power of small changes!

As we navigate the world of exercise and diabetes management, remember that consistency is key. ⬜⬜ Start small, stay committed, and gradually build up your exercise routine over time. Listen to your body, be patient with yourself, and celebrate your progress along the way. ⬜⬜

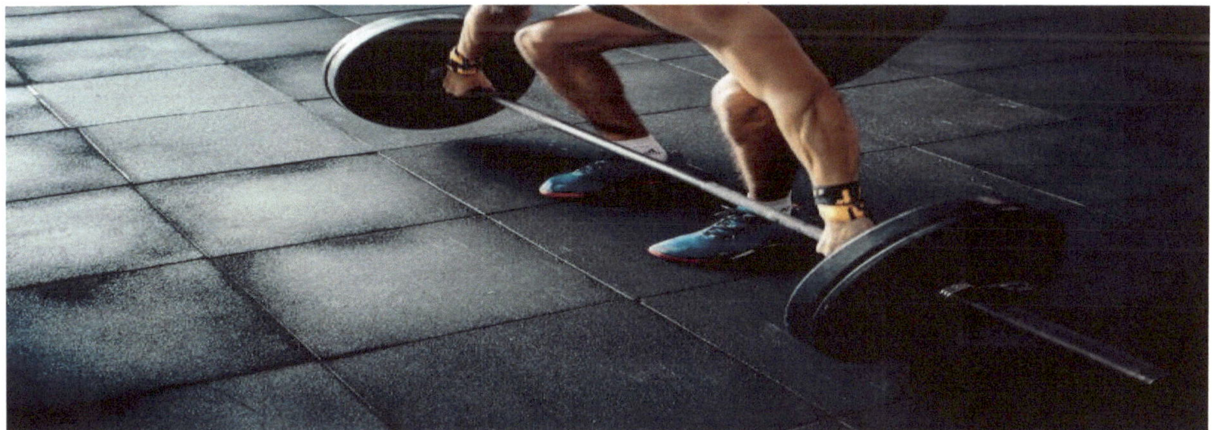

10 Action Points

1. **Set SMART Fitness Goals**: Establish specific, measurable, achievable, relevant, and time-bound goals for your exercise routine to keep you motivated and focused.
2. **Find Activities You Enjoy**: Explore different types of physical activities, such as walking, cycling, swimming, yoga, or dancing, and choose ones that you genuinely enjoy to make exercise a sustainable part of your lifestyle.
3. **Schedule Regular Workouts**: Block out dedicated time in your schedule for exercise sessions and treat them as non-negotiable appointments with yourself.
4. **Mix Up Your Routine:** Incorporate a variety of workouts into your routine, including cardio, strength training, flexibility exercises, and balance work, to keep things interesting and challenge different muscle groups.
5. **Find Accountability Partners:** Recruit friends, family members, or workout buddies to join you in your fitness journey and hold each other accountable for sticking to your exercise goals.
6. **Start Slow and Gradually Increase Intensity:** If you're new to exercise or returning after a break, start with low-intensity activities and gradually increase the duration and intensity of your workouts as your fitness level improves.
7. **Listen to Your Body:** Pay attention to how your body feels during exercise and adjust your intensity or duration as needed to avoid injury and prevent burnout.
8. **Incorporate Movement Throughout the Day:** Look for opportunities to increase your daily movement by taking the stairs instead of the elevator, walking or biking instead of driving, and incorporating more activity breaks into your workday.
9. **Stay Hydrated and Fuel Your Body Properly**: Drink plenty of water before, during, and after exercise to stay hydrated, and fuel your body with balanced meals and snacks that provide the energy you need for your workouts.
10. **Celebrate Your Progress**: Recognize and celebrate your achievements, whether it's completing a challenging workout, reaching a fitness milestone, or sticking to your exercise routine consistently. Acknowledging your progress will help keep you motivated and inspired to continue moving forward on your fitness journey.

Chapter 5:
Sleep and its impact on Diabetes and Weight loss

Importance of Sleep in Diabetes Control

Sleep isn't just a time to recharge your batteries—it's a critical component of overall health and well-being. Yet, in today's fast-paced world, sleep is often sacrificed in favour of work, social commitments, and screen time. But here's the catch: skimping on sleep can have serious consequences for your health, including increased risk of obesity, insulin resistance, and type 2 diabetes. □Sleep deprivation disrupts hormonal balance, increases appetite, and impairs glucose metabolism. From the release of hunger hormones like ghrelin to the suppression of satiety hormones like leptin, sleep influences hunger, cravings, and food choices. □□Establishing healthy bedtime routines, and addressing common sleep disruptions such as stress, anxiety, and sleep disorders. From creating a relaxing bedtime ritual to setting a consistent sleep schedule and minimizing exposure to electronic devices before bedtime, we'll provide you with a roadmap to better sleep. Whether it's a morning jog, an afternoon yoga class, or an evening stroll, incorporating exercise into your daily routine can promote deeper, more restorative sleep. And let's not forget about the power of mindfulness and relaxation techniques in promoting sleep. From deep breathing exercises and progressive muscle relaxation to guided imagery and meditation.

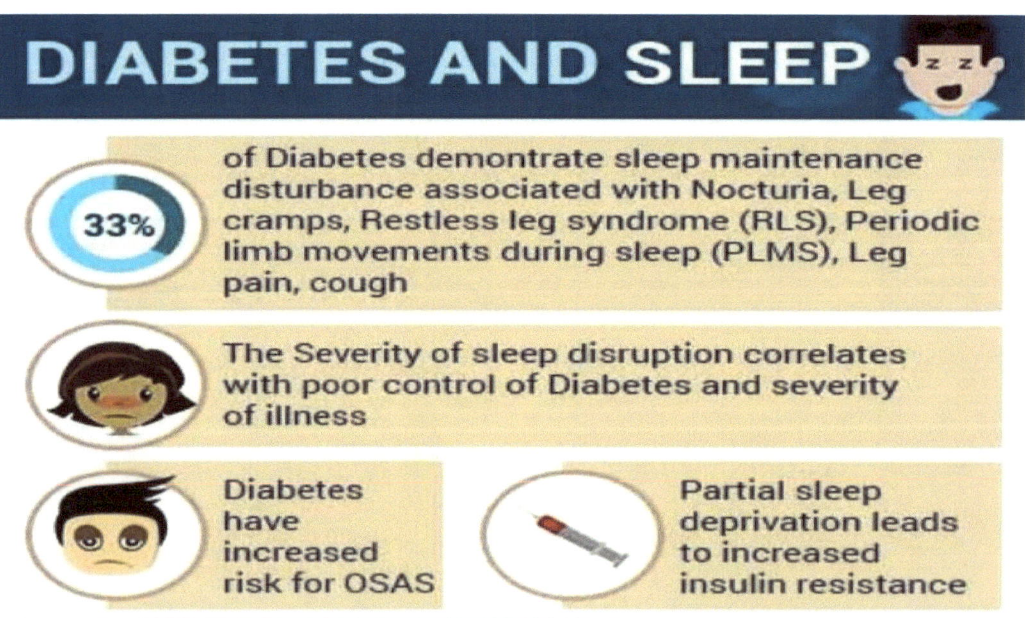

10 Action Points

1. **Establish a Consistent Sleep Schedule:** Set a regular bedtime and wake-up time, even on weekends, to regulate your body's internal clock and improve sleep quality.
2. **Create a Relaxing Bedtime Routine:** Develop a calming bedtime ritual to signal to your body that it's time to wind down. This could include activities such as reading, taking a warm bath, or practicing relaxation techniques like deep breathing or meditation.
3. **Optimize Your Sleep Environment:** Make your bedroom conducive to sleep by keeping it cool, dark, and quiet. Invest in comfortable bedding, block out external noise with earplugs or white noise machines, and use blackout curtains to minimize light exposure.
4. **Limit Screen Time Before Bed:** Reduce exposure to electronic devices such as smartphones, tablets, and computers in the hour leading up to bedtime, as the blue light emitted from screens can disrupt the production of melatonin and interfere with sleep.
5. **Watch Your Caffeine Intake:** Limit consumption of caffeine, especially in the afternoon and evening, as it can interfere with sleep quality and disrupt your natural sleep-wake cycle.
6. **Practice Stress Reduction Techniques:** Incorporate relaxation techniques such as deep breathing exercises, progressive muscle relaxation into your bedtime routine to calm the mind and prepare for sleep.
7. **Stay Active During the Day:** Engage in regular physical activity throughout the day to promote deeper, more restorative sleep at night. Aim for at least 30 minutes of moderate-intensity exercise most days of the week.
8. **Monitor Your Sleep Patterns:** Keep track of your sleep patterns and habits using a sleep diary or tracking device to identify trends, track improvements, and make adjustments to your sleep routine as needed.
9. **Limit Naps During the Day:** Avoid long or late afternoon naps, as they can interfere with your ability to fall asleep at night and disrupt your sleep cycle.
10. **Seek Professional Help if Needed:** If you're struggling with chronic sleep issues or sleep disorders such as insomnia or sleep apnea, don't hesitate to seek help from a healthcare professional who can provide guidance, evaluation, and treatment options tailored to your individual needs.

Chapter 6: Social Support for Diabetes Reversal

The Power of Social Support

Imagine embarking on a health journey with a tribe of like-minded individuals cheering you on every step of the way—**a network of friends, family, and peers** who lift you up, inspire you, and hold you accountable to your goals. This is the power of social support—a force that can propel you towards success and transform your health from the inside out. □□From reducing stress levels and boosting mood to improving adherence to healthy habits and enhancing self-efficacy, social support serves as a cornerstone of success in managing diabetes and achieving weight loss goals. It's the invisible hand guiding you towards a healthier, happier life. □□But social support isn't just about receiving—it's also about giving. By being part of a community, you have the opportunity to offer encouragement, inspiration, and wisdom to others on their health journey. Whether it's sharing your own experiences, offering words of encouragement, or celebrating the successes of fellow community members, your contributions can make a world of difference to those around you. It's a beautiful cycle of support and reciprocity that strengthens bonds and fosters a sense of belonging. □□From joining online forums and social media groups to participating in local support groups, wellness workshops, or exercise classes, there are countless avenues for connecting with others who share your health goals and aspirations. It's about finding your tribe—your tribe of kindred spirits who lift you up, inspire you, and walk alongside you on your journey towards better health. □□

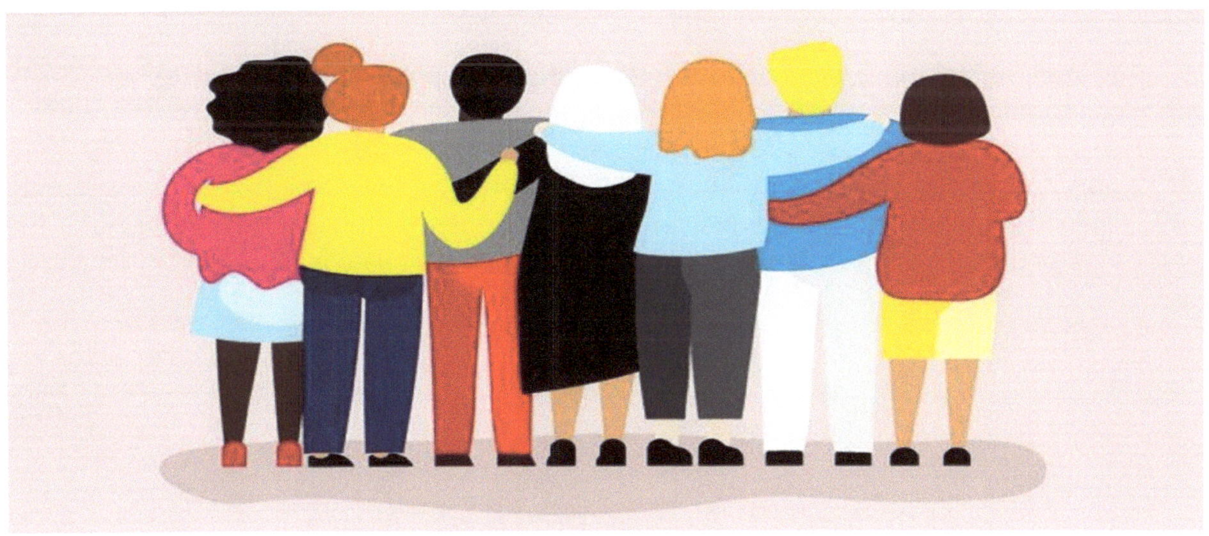

10 Action Points:

1. **Join a Support Group:** Seek out local or online support groups focused on diabetes management and weight loss to connect with others who share similar health goals and experiences.
2. **Participate in Community Events:** Attend wellness workshops, fitness classes, or health-related events in your community to meet like-minded individuals and build your support network.
3. **Engage on Social media:** Join social media groups or online forums dedicated to health and wellness where you can interact with others, share resources, and receive support and encouragement.
4. **Attend Wellness Workshops:** Take advantage of workshops or seminars focused on topics such as nutrition, exercise, stress management, and mindfulness to learn new skills and connect with others on their health journey.
5. **Volunteer in Your Community:** Get involved in local volunteering opportunities related to health and wellness initiatives to connect with others while giving back to your community.
6. **Start a Walking Group:** Organize a regular walking group with friends, family, or coworkers to enjoy physical activity together while providing social support and accountability.
7. **Host Healthy Potlucks or Cooking Nights:** Invite friends or family members to participate in healthy potlucks or cooking nights where you can share nutritious recipes, cooking tips, and support each other's dietary goals.
8. **Seek Out a Health Coach or Mentor:** Consider working with a health coach or mentor who can provide personalized support, guidance, and accountability on your health journey.
9. **Attend Supportive Events or Retreats:** Look for wellness retreats, health expos, or educational events focused on diabetes management and weight loss where you can connect with experts and fellow participants in a supportive environment.
10. **Stay Connected with Loved Ones:** Foster meaningful connections with friends, family members, and loved ones by regularly reaching out, scheduling quality time together, and engaging in open and supportive conversations about your health goals and challenges.

Chapter 7: The Role of Yoga & Meditation in Diabetes Reversal

Understanding the Mind Body Connection

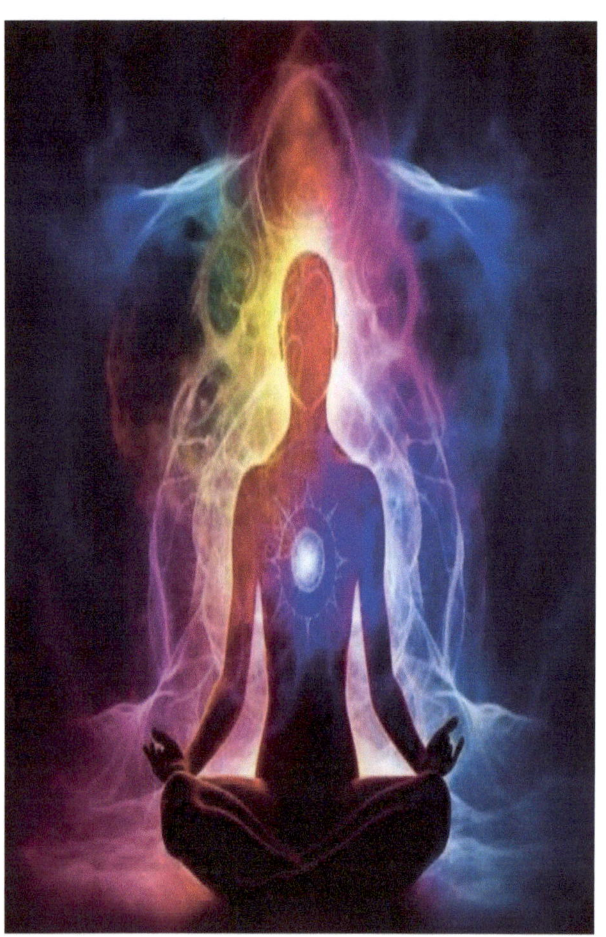

Understanding the mind-body connection is crucial for adults with type 2 diabetes on their journey towards diabetes reversal. The mind and body are intricately connected, and the way we think and feel can have a significant impact on our physical health. Research has shown that stress, anxiety, and negative emotions can worsen diabetes symptoms and make it harder to manage blood sugar levels. By understanding this connection, individuals can learn to harness the power of their mind to support their body in achieving optimal health.

When we are stressed or anxious, our bodies release hormones like **cortisol** and **adrenaline**, which can raise blood sugar levels and make it harder for insulin to regulate glucose. This can lead to spikes in blood sugar levels and ultimately worsen diabetes symptoms. By practicing mindfulness techniques such as meditation, deep breathing, and visualization, individuals can learn to calm their minds and reduce stress levels, which in turn can help to improve blood sugar control and overall health.

In addition to reducing stress, mindfulness practices can also help individuals with type 2 diabetes to develop a greater awareness of their bodies and their needs. By tuning in to their bodies, individuals can become more attuned to signals of hunger, satiety, and cravings, which can help them make healthier food choices and maintain a balanced diet. Mindfulness can also help individuals to listen to their bodies and recognize when they are feeling tired or in need of rest, allowing them to prioritize self-care and prevent burnout.

In conclusion, understanding the mind-body connection is essential for adults with type 2 diabetes who are seeking to reverse their condition through a combination of medication and meditation. By recognizing the impact of stress and emotions on physical health, practicing mindfulness techniques, and adopting a positive mindset, individuals can support their bodies in achieving optimal health and well-being. Through the power of the mind-body connection, individuals with type 2 diabetes can take control of their health, improve blood sugar control, and ultimately reverse their diabetes.

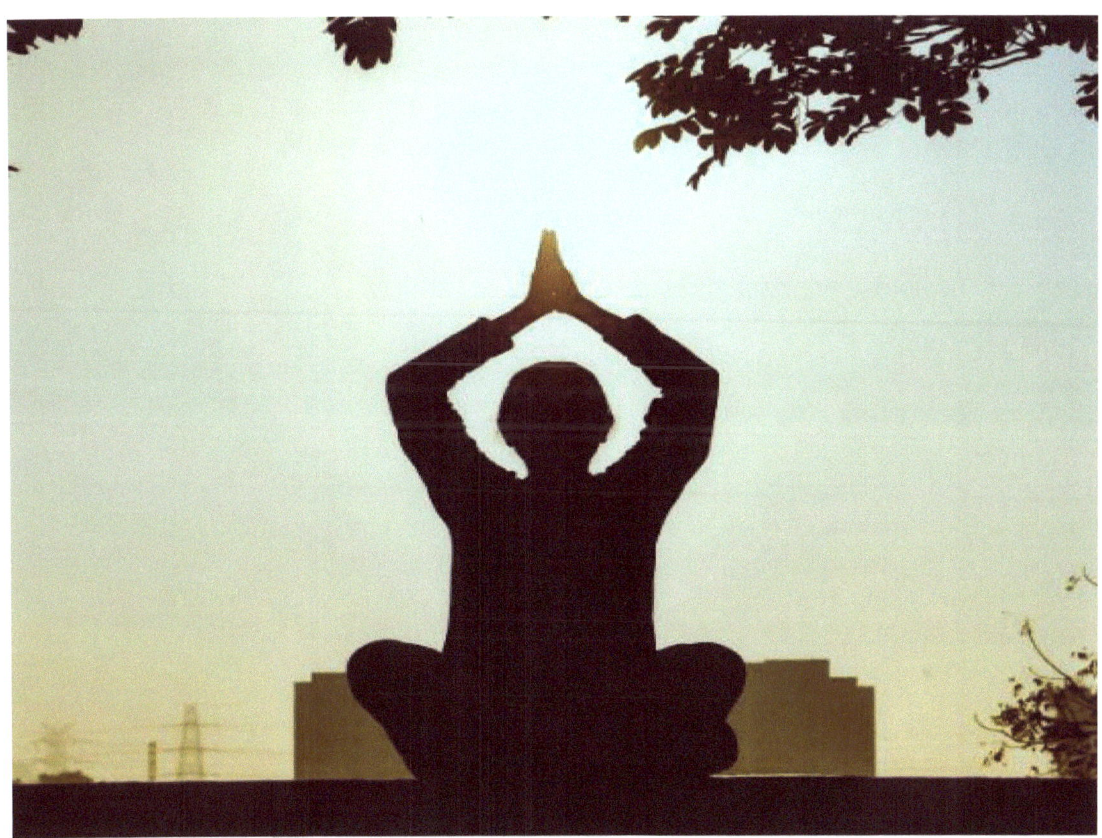

Benefits of Meditation for Diabetes Management

Meditation has been shown to be a powerful tool in managing diabetes. By incorporating meditation into your daily routine, you can experience a wide range of benefits that can help improve your overall health and well-being. One of the key benefits of meditation for diabetes management is **stress reduction**. Stress has been linked to the development and progression of diabetes. Meditation can help lower stress levels, which in turn can help improve blood sugar control and reduce the risk of complications.

In addition to reducing stress, meditation can also help **improve insulin sensitivity**. Insulin sensitivity is the body's ability to respond to and utilize insulin effectively. By practicing meditation regularly, you can help improve your body's sensitivity to insulin, which can lead to better blood sugar control. This can help reduce the need for medication and lower the risk of complications associated with diabetes.

Another benefit of meditation for diabetes management is its ability to promote **mindfulness**. Mindfulness involves being present in the moment and fully aware of your thoughts, feelings, and sensations. By practicing mindfulness through meditation, you can become more in tune with your body and its needs. This can help you make healthier choices when it comes to managing your diabetes, such as eating a balanced diet and getting regular exercise.

Meditation can also help improve **sleep quality**, which is important for those with diabetes. Poor sleep can have a negative impact on blood sugar control and overall health. By practicing meditation before bed, you can help relax your mind and body, making it easier to fall asleep and stay asleep throughout the night. This can lead to better blood sugar control and improved overall health.

Overall, incorporating meditation into your diabetes management plan can have a positive impact on your health and wellbeing. By reducing stress, improving insulin sensitivity, promoting mindfulness, and enhancing sleep quality, meditation can help you better manage your diabetes and live a healthier, happier life. Consider adding meditation to your daily routine and experience the benefits for yourself.

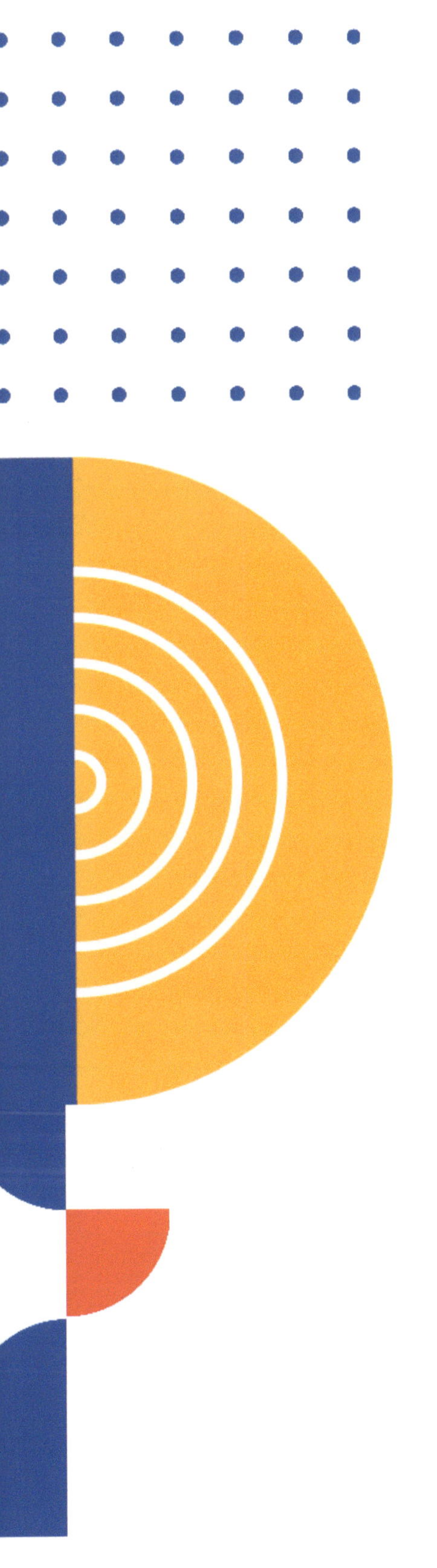

Different Types of Meditation Practices

Meditation is a powerful tool that can benefit adults with type2 diabetes in managing their condition and improving their overall health. There are various types of meditation practices that can be incorporated into daily routines to help reduce stress, improve mental clarity, and promote emotional well- being.

One type of meditation practice that is commonly used by adults with type 2 diabetes is **mindfulness meditation**. This practice involves focusing on the present moment and being aware of thoughts, feelings, and sensations without judgment. Mindfulness meditation can help individuals manage stress, anxiety, and depression, all of which are common comorbidities of type 2 diabetes. By practicing mindfulness meditation regularly, individuals can cultivate a sense of inner peace and calm that can positively impact their physical and mental health.

Another popular meditation practice for adults with type 2 diabetes is **loving-kindness meditation.** This practice involves cultivating feelings of love, compassion, and kindness towards oneself and others. Loving-kindness meditation can help individuals develop a positive mindset and improve their relationships with others, which can have a beneficial impact on their overall well-being. By practicing loving-kindness meditation regularly, individuals can foster a sense of gratitude and appreciation for life, which can help them cope with the challenges of living with type 2 diabetes.

Body scan meditation is another type of meditation practice that can be beneficial for adults with type 2 diabetes. This practice involves focusing on different parts of the body and bringing awareness to any sensations or tensions that may be present. Body scan meditation can help individuals relax their muscles, release tension, and improve their overall physical comfort.

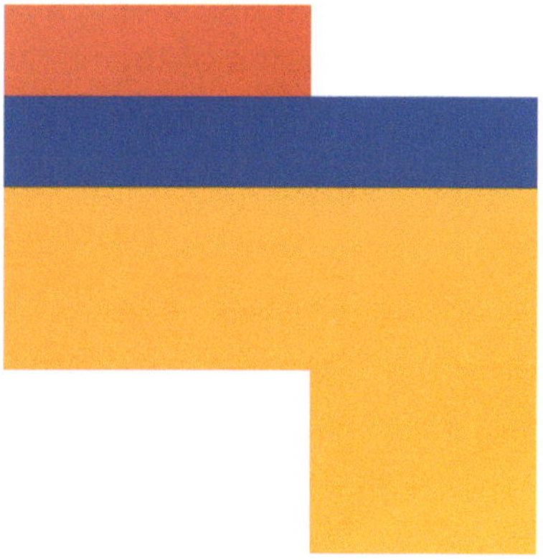

Best Yoga Poses for Diabetes Reversal:

In type 2 diabetes **yoga asanas** directly stimulate the pancreas and simultaneously reduce stress levels, leading to decreased blood sugar levels and fewer associated complications. Additionally, yoga's relaxation techniques help lower cortisol, a stress hormone, which has a positive impact on blood pressure and blood sugar levels.

1. **Surya Namaskar (Sun Salutation):**
   One of the greatest asanas for diabetes, it includes 12 postures carried out in a smooth, continuous sequence. Regular Sun Salutation practice can boost your vitality and general physical and mental well-being.

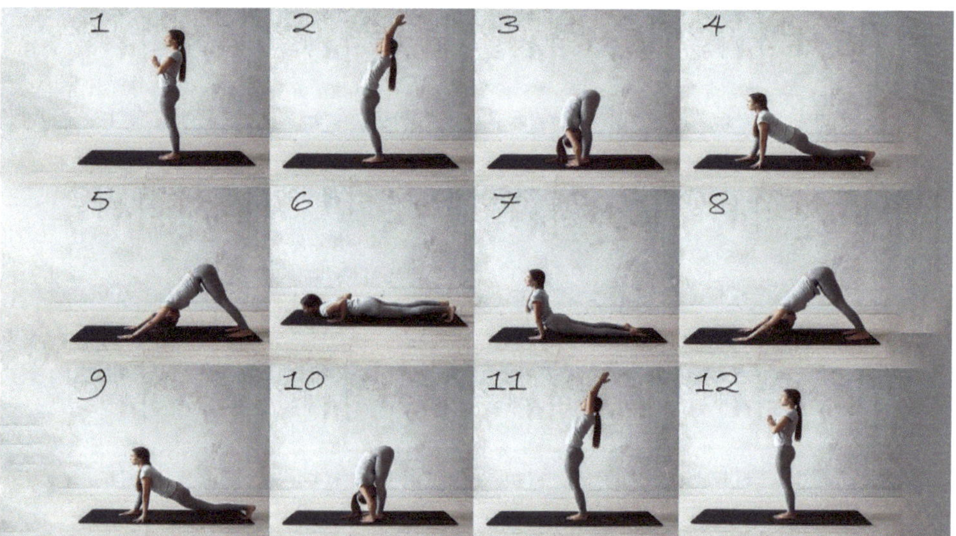

The Sun Salutation, also known as Surya Namaskar, has a number of benefits, including the stimulation of the respiratory and digestive systems, efficient muscle and joint warm-up, increased circulation and flexibility, and improved general body awareness and concentration.

2. Viparita Karani (Legs Up the Wall Pose):

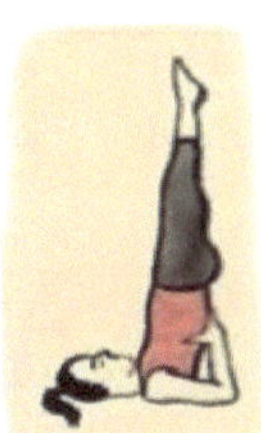

This gentle pose involves lying on your back with your legs extended upward against a wall. It only takes a few minutes a day and can leave you feeling refreshed and rejuvenated. Practicing this pose can help you relax and reduce stress levels, as well as relieve headaches and boost your energy. This Yoga targets the legs, hips, and lower back muscles.

3. Bhujangasana (Cobra Stretch):

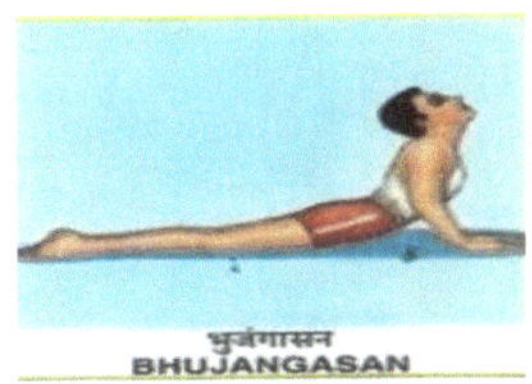

Bhujangasana also known as the Cobra Stretch is an easy yoga pose that stimulates the pancreas and simultaneously reduce stress levels, leading to decreased blood sugar level also enhances the strength of the spine, arms, and shoulders, and improves posture and alignment. To do this pose lie on your stomach and place your hands on the floor near your chest. Gently lift your shoulders and upper body. Make sure to bend your elbows slightly. Hold this asana for up to 30 seconds.

4. Adho Mukha Svanasana (Downward Dog):

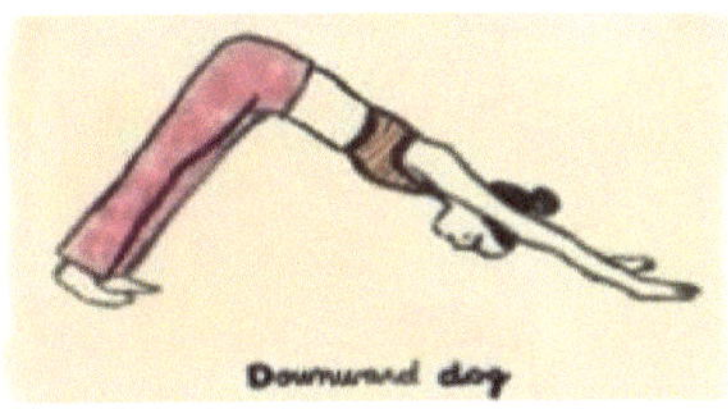

The Downward-facing Dog Pose in yoga can enhance blood circulation and improve insulin sensitivity, making it beneficial for those with diabetes. Begin on hands and knees and lift your hips to form an inverted V-shape. This pose can also increase muscular strength and core stability, lower blood pressure, and improve overall circulation.

5. Phalakasana (Plank Pose):

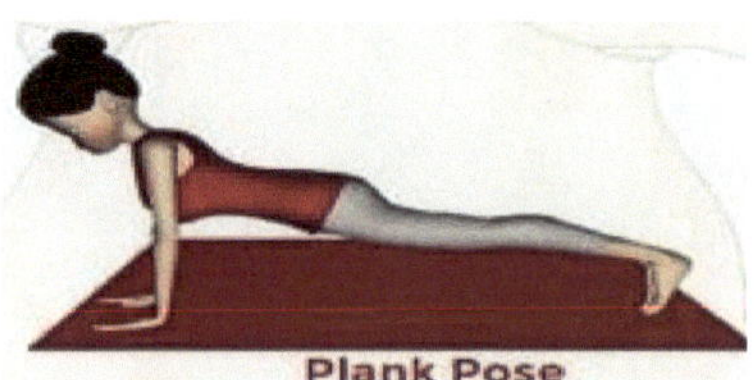

The Plank Pose, or Phalakasana, is a demanding yoga pose, especially beneficial for managing diabetes. Regular practice of the Plank Pose not only establishes a solid foundation for advanced yoga postures but also enhances overall physical fitness.

6. Mandukasana (Frog's Pose):

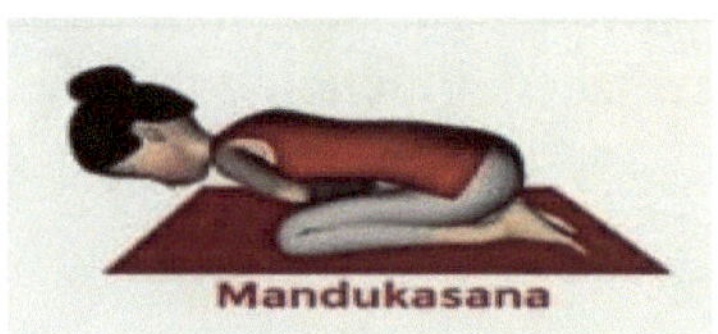

Frog pose Increases the quantity of insulin so it is beneficial for curing diabetes.
- Sit in Vajrasana pose.
- Place your right palm on your left palm; keep them on the navel.
- Now press your stomach inwards.
- Exhale and bend forward (same as method 1), and keep looking straight.
- Hold your breath and position for some time.
- Slowly inhale and come back to Starting Position.
- Repeat this 3 to 4 times.

7. Balasana (Child's Pose):

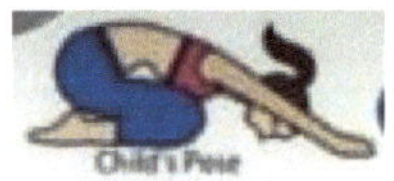

This reclining position increases relaxation, which may support the growth of beta cells that produce insulin. Additionally, it might aid in reducing anxiety, fatigue, and back and neck problems.

8. Dhanurasana (Bow Pose):

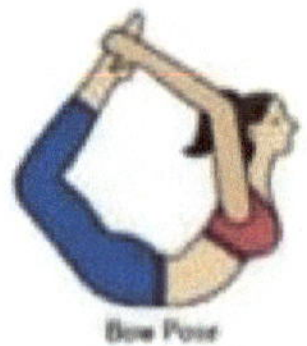

This backbend posture not only expands the chest but also activates the abdominal organs, potentially aiding in blood sugar regulation and alleviating issues like constipation and respiratory ailments.

Now, you may easily understand how yoga can help with diabetes management by doing these positions. If you currently have this medical condition, learning the technique and practice of yoga will enable you to significantly lessen the symptoms & medications. With a trainer's assistance, you can begin with as little as two or three days per week and then build up as your body requires.

In conclusion, there are various types of meditation practices and yoga poses that can benefit adults with type 2 diabetes in managing their condition and improving their overall health. Mindfulness meditation, loving-kindness meditation, and body scan meditation are just a few examples of the many meditation practices available. By exploring different types of meditation practices and finding the one that resonates with them, individuals with type 2 diabetes can experience the numerous benefits that meditation has to offer. Whether it's reducing stress, improving mental clarity, or promoting emotional wellbeing, meditation can be a valuable tool in the journey towards diabetes reversal and overall wellbeing.

Chapter 8: Creating a Diabetes Reversal Plan

Setting Realistic Goals

Setting realistic goals is a crucial step in the journey towards diabetes reversal. As adults with type 2 diabetes, it is important to understand that achieving optimal health is a gradual process that requires dedication and commitment. By setting realistic goals, you can create a roadmap for success and track your progress along the way.

When it comes to setting goals for diabetes reversal, it is important to be specific and measurable. Instead of setting a vague goal like "I want to lower my blood sugar levels," try setting a specific target, such as **"I want to lower my fasting blood sugar levels by 20 points within the next three months."** This way, you have a clear target to aim for and can track your progress over time.

It is also important to set achievable goals that are within your control. While it is great to have ambitious goals, setting unrealistic targets can set you up for disappointment and frustration. Instead, focus on small, manageable steps that you can take each day to work towards your larger goal of diabetes reversal.

In addition to setting specific and achievable goals, it is important to set a timeline for achieving them. By setting deadlines for your goals, you create a sense of urgency and motivation to stay on track. Whether you are aiming to lose a certain amount of weight, improve your A1C levels, or incorporate more physical activity into your routine, having a timeline can help you stay focused and accountable.

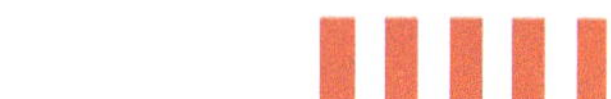

Remember, setting realistic goals is not about perfection, but progress. Celebrate your successes along the way, no matter how small they may seem. By setting realistic goals and staying committed to your journey towards diabetes reversal, you can take control of your health and improve your overall wellbeing.

Nutrition and Meal Planning

Proper nutrition and meal planning are essential components of managing and potentially reversing type 2 diabetes.

By making healthy food choices and creating a balanced meal plan, individuals with diabetes can better control their blood sugar levels and improve their overall health. It is important to focus on consuming a variety of nutrient-dense foods such as fruits, vegetables, whole grains, lean proteins, and healthy fats.

When planning meals, it is crucial to consider the **glycemic index** of foods. The glycemic index measures how quickly a food raises blood sugar levels. Foods with a high glycemic index can cause spikes in blood sugar, which can be detrimental for individuals with diabetes. It is recommended to choose foods with a low to moderate glycemic index to help maintain stable blood sugar levels throughout the day.

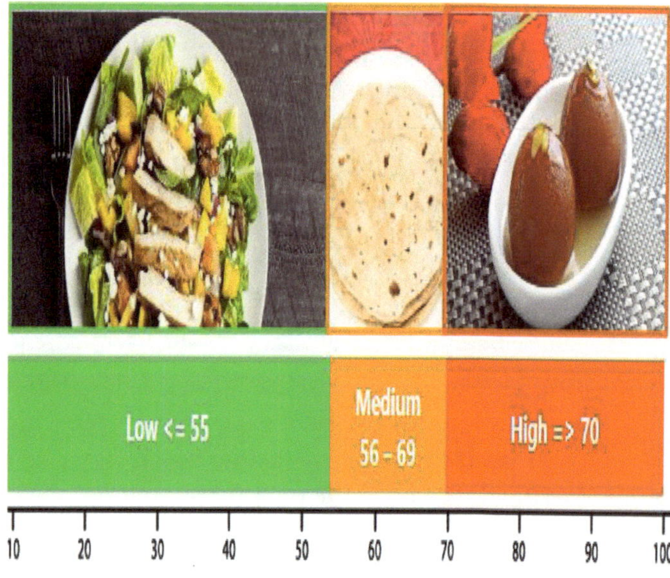

In addition to the glycemic index, **portion control** is another important aspect of meal planning for individuals with type 2 diabetes. Eating the right portion sizes can help prevent overeating and regulate blood sugar levels. It is advisable to use measuring cups or a food scale to accurately portion out meals and snacks. By practicing portion control, individuals can better manage their weight and improve their diabetes management.

Another key consideration for nutrition and meal planning is to limit the intake of processed and sugary foods. These types of foods can lead to unstable blood sugar levels and contribute to weight gain, both of which can worsen diabetes symptoms. Instead, focus on whole, unprocessed foods that are rich in vitamins, minerals, and antioxidants. By making healthier food choices, individuals can positively impact their diabetes management and overall well-being.

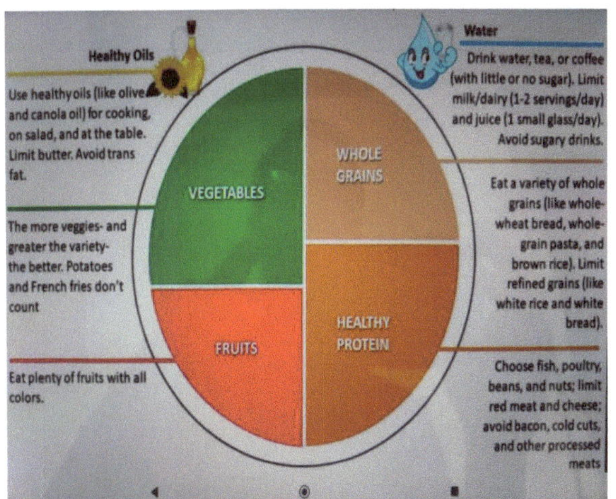

Overall, proper nutrition and meal planning play a crucial role in reversing type 2 diabetes. By focusing on nutrient-dense foods, the glycemic index, portion control, and limiting processed foods, individuals can better control their blood sugar levels and improve their quality of life. It is important to work with a healthcare provider or nutritionist to create a personalized meal plan that fits individual needs and preferences. With dedication and commitment to making healthy choices, individuals with type 2 diabetes can achieve better health outcomes and potentially reverse their diabetes.

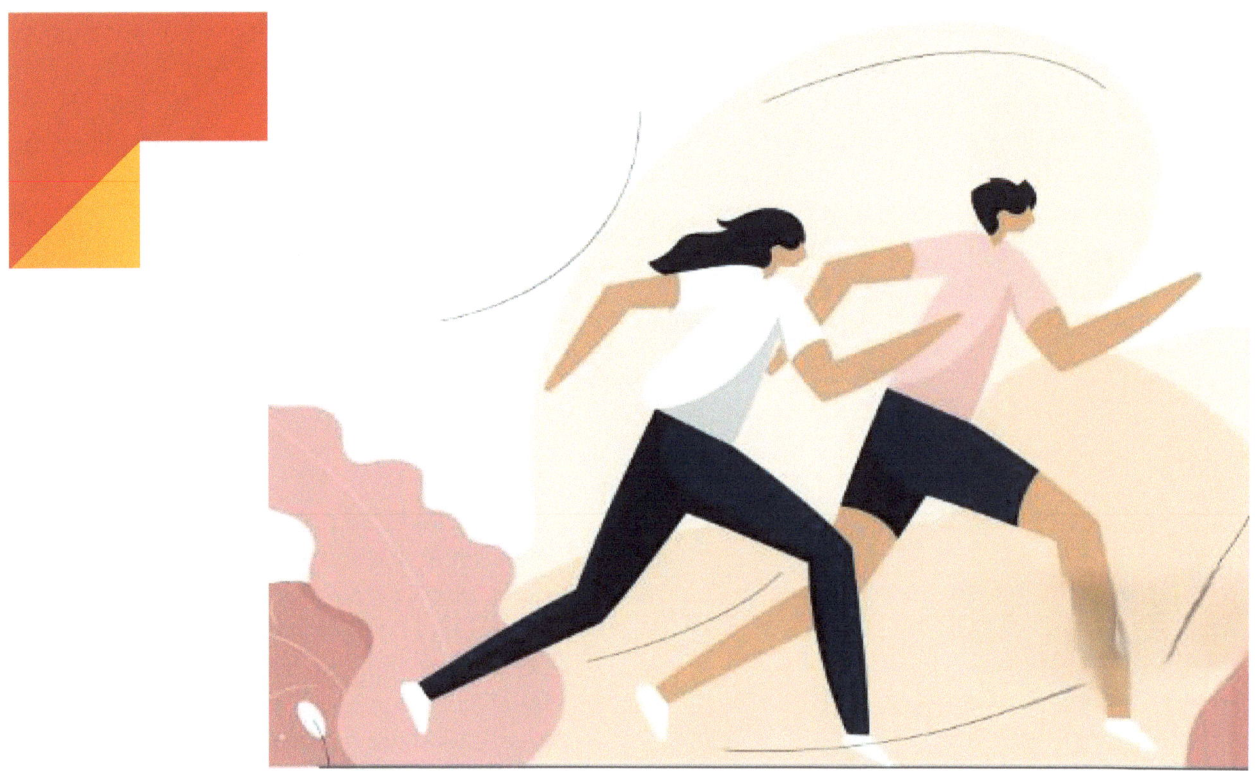

Incorporating Exercise into Your Routine

Incorporating regular exercise into your daily routine is an essential component of managing and even reversing type 2 diabetes. Exercise can help improve insulin sensitivity, lower blood sugar levels, and reduce the risk of complications associated with diabetes. It is important to find an exercise regimen that works for you and fits into your lifestyle. Whether it's walking, swimming, cycling, or yoga, finding an activity that you enjoy will make it easier to stick to a regular exercise routine.

One of the key benefits of exercise for individuals with type 2 diabetes is its ability to help control weight. Maintaining a healthy weight is crucial for managing diabetes as excess weight can lead to insulin resistance and higher blood sugar levels. By incorporating regular physical activity into your routine, you can help shed excess pounds and improve your overall health. Aim for at least 150 minutes of moderate- intensity exercise per week, spread out over several days.

In addition to weight management, exercise can also help reduce stress levels and improve mental health. Living with diabetes can be stressful, and exercise can be a great way to relieve tension and improve your mood. Physical activity releases endorphins, which are natural mood boosters, and can help alleviate symptoms of anxiety and depression. Incorporating exercise into your routine can have a positive impact on both your physical and mental wel-being. When starting an exercise regimen, it is important to consult with your healthcare provider to ensure that you are engaging in safe and appropriate activities. Your doctor can help you determine the best type and intensity of exercise for your individual needs and health goals. They can also provide guidance on monitoring your blood sugar levels before, during, and after exercise to ensure that you are staying within a safe range. By working closely with your healthcare team, you can create a **personalized exercise plan** that will help you manage your diabetes effectively.

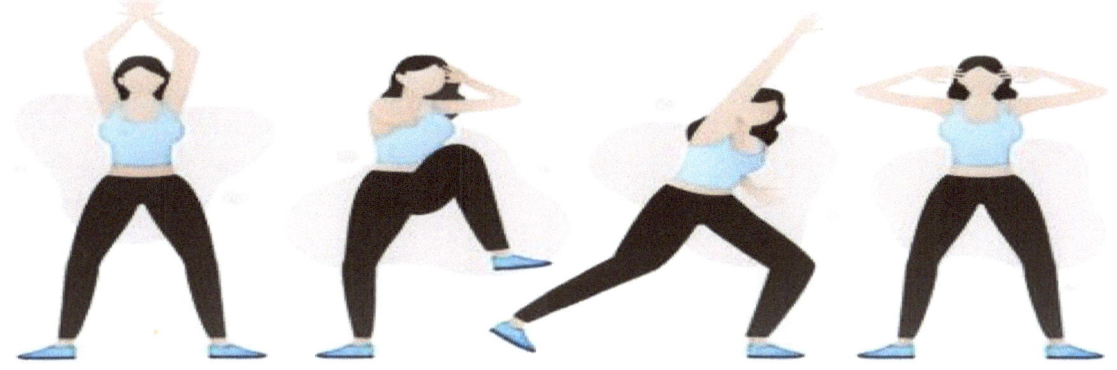

In conclusion, incorporating exercise into your daily routine is a powerful tool for managing type 2 diabetes and improving overall health. By finding an activity that you enjoy and fits into your lifestyle, you can make exercise a regular part of your self-care routine. Whether it's going for a walk, taking a yoga class, or hitting the gym, finding ways to move your body regularly can have a significant impact on your diabetes management. Remember to consult with your healthcare provider before starting any new exercise program and to monitor your blood sugar levels to ensure that you are exercising safely and effectively. With dedication and commitment, you can harness the benefits of exercise to help reverse your diabetes and improve your quality of life.

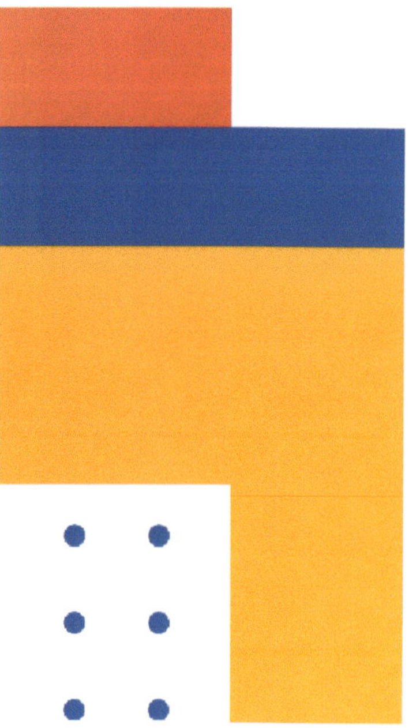

Chapter 9 Implementing Lifestyle Changes for Diabetes Reversal

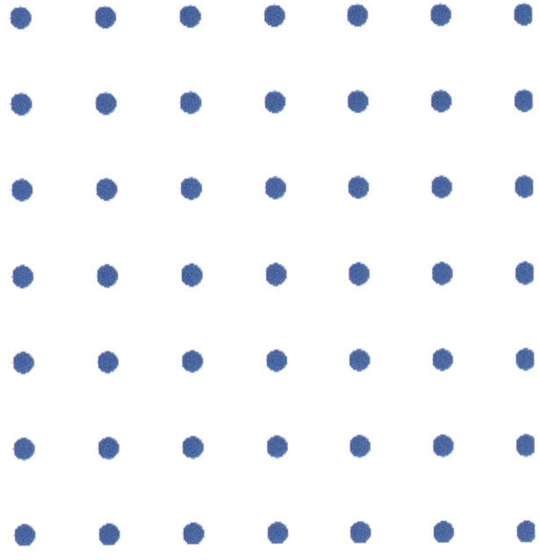

Stress Management Techniques

Stress can have a significant impact on our overall health, especially for adults with type 2 diabetes. When we are stressed, our bodies release hormones that can raise blood sugar levels and make it harder to manage diabetes effectively. Therefore, learning how to manage stress is essential for diabetes reversal. Here are some stress management techniques that can help you take control of your stress levels and improve your diabetes management.

One effective stress management technique is **mindfulness meditation**. This practice involves focusing on the present moment and accepting it without judgment. By practicing mindfulness meditation regularly, you can train your mind to be more aware of your thoughts and emotions, which can help you respond to stress in a more calm and thoughtful manner. This can lead to lower stress levels and better diabetes management over time.

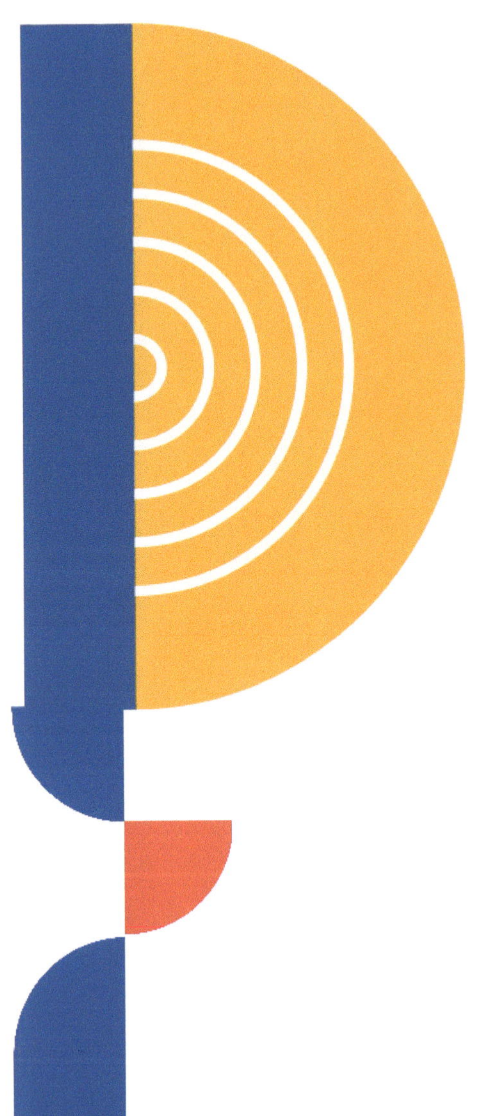

Another helpful stress management technique is **deep breathing exercises**. When we are stressed, our breathing tends to become shallow and rapid, which can exacerbate feelings of anxiety and stress. By practicing deep breathing exercises, you can slow down your breathing and activate your body's relaxation response, leading to reduced stress levels and improved overall wellbeing. Deep breathing exercises can be done anywhere, making them a convenient and effective tool for managing stress on the go.

Regular physical activity is another excellent way to manage stress and improve diabetes management. Exercise releases endorphins, which are chemicals in the brain that act as natural painkillers and mood elevators. By incorporating regular physical activity into your routine, you can reduce stress levels, improve your mood, and enhance your overall health.

Aim for at least **30 minutes** of moderate-intensity exercise most days of the week to experience the stress-relieving benefits of physical activity. In addition to mindfulness meditation, deep breathing exercises, and regular physical activity, it's essential to prioritize self-care as part of your stress management routine. This can include activities such as spending time with loved ones, engaging in hobbies you enjoy, getting enough sleep, and eating a balanced diet. Taking care of yourself can help you feel more resilient in the face of stress and better equipped to manage your diabetes effectively.

In conclusion, managing stress is crucial for adults with type 2 diabetes looking to reverse their condition. By incorporating stress management techniques such as **mindfulness meditation, deep breathing exercises, regular physical activity, and self-care into your routine**,
you can reduce stress levels, improve your diabetes management, and enhance your overall wellbeing. Experiment with these techniques to find what works best for you, and remember that managing stress is a lifelong journey that requires practice and patience.

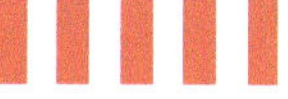

Sleep Hygiene and Diabetes Control

Sleep hygiene plays a crucial role in managing diabetes effectively. For adults with type 2 diabetes, maintaining good sleep habits can significantly impact blood sugar levels and overall health. Research has shown that poor sleep quality and inadequate sleep duration can lead to insulin resistance, weight gain, and difficulty in controlling blood sugar levels. Therefore, it is essential to prioritize sleep hygiene as part of your diabetes management plan.

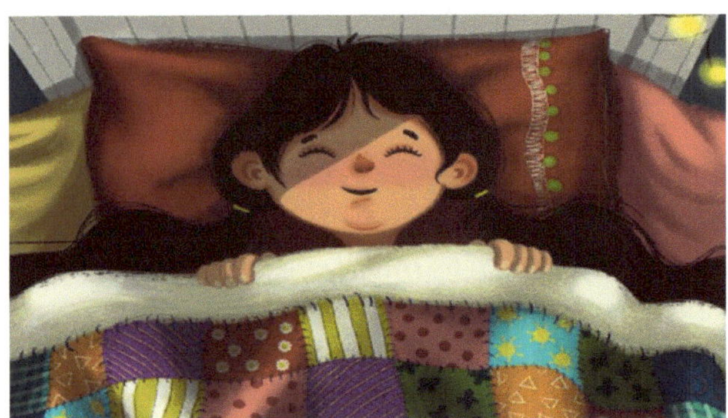

Creating a relaxing bedtime routine can also promote better sleep quality for adults with type 2 diabetes. Engaging in calming activities before bed, such as **reading, meditating, or taking a warm bath**, can help signal to your body that it is time to wind down and prepare for sleep. **Avoiding** stimulating activities, such as **watching TV or using electronic devices**, close to bedtime can also improve your ability to fall asleep and stay asleep throughout the night.

It is important to create a sleep-friendly environment. Keep your **bedroom dark, quiet, and cool** to promote restful sleep. Investing in a comfortable mattress and pillows can also improve your sleep quality and overall comfort. For adults with type 2 diabetes, optimizing your sleep environment can help reduce stress, improve blood sugar control, and enhance overall well-being.

Social Support &
Accountability

Social support and accountability are crucial components in the journey towards reversing type 2 diabetes. Having a strong support system can make all the difference in staying motivated and on track with your health goals. Whether it's family, friends, or a support group, surrounding yourself with people who understand and encourage your efforts can be immensely helpful.

One way to harness the power of social support is to join a diabetes reversal support group. These groups provide a safe space for individuals with type 2 diabetes to share their experiences, struggles, and successes. Being able to connect with others who are going through similar challenges can be incredibly validating and empowering. It also provides an opportunity to learn from others and gain new insights into managing and reversing diabetes.

In addition to social support, accountability is another key factor in achieving success in reversing type 2 diabetes. Being held accountable to someone, whether it's a friend, family member, or healthcare provider, can help keep you accountable to your health goals. Knowing that someone is checking in on your progress can provide an extra layer of motivation to stay committed to making positive changes in your lifestyle.

One effective way to stay accountable is to set specific goals and regularly track your progress. This could include monitoring your blood sugar levels, tracking your physical activity, or keeping a food diary. By setting clear and achievable goals, you can measure your progress and make adjustments as needed to stay on track towards reversing your diabetes.

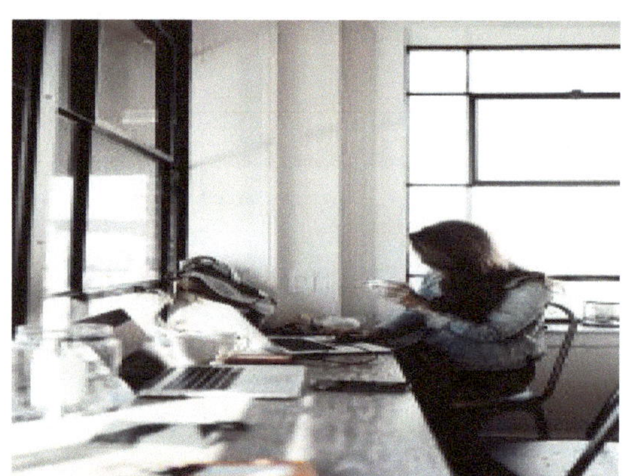

Remember, you are not alone in your journey to reverse type 2 diabetes. By building a strong support system and holding yourself accountable to your health goals, you can increase your chances of success and improve your overall wel-being. Embrace the power of social support and accountability as you work towards achieving optimal health and reversing your diabetes.

Chapter 10:
Monitoring Progress and Adjusting Your Plan

Tracking Blood Sugar Levels

Tracking your blood sugar levels is a crucial aspect of managing and reversing Type 2 diabetes. By monitoring your blood sugar regularly, you can gain valuable insights into how your body responds to different foods, activities, and medications. This information can help you make informed decisions about your diet, exercise routine, and overall lifestyle choices to better control your blood sugar levels. To effectively track your blood sugar levels, it is essential to invest in a reliable blood glucose monitor. These devices are easy to use and provide accurate readings of your blood sugar levels at any given time. By regularly checking your blood sugar levels throughout the day, you can identify patterns and trends that may indicate how well you are managing your diabetes.

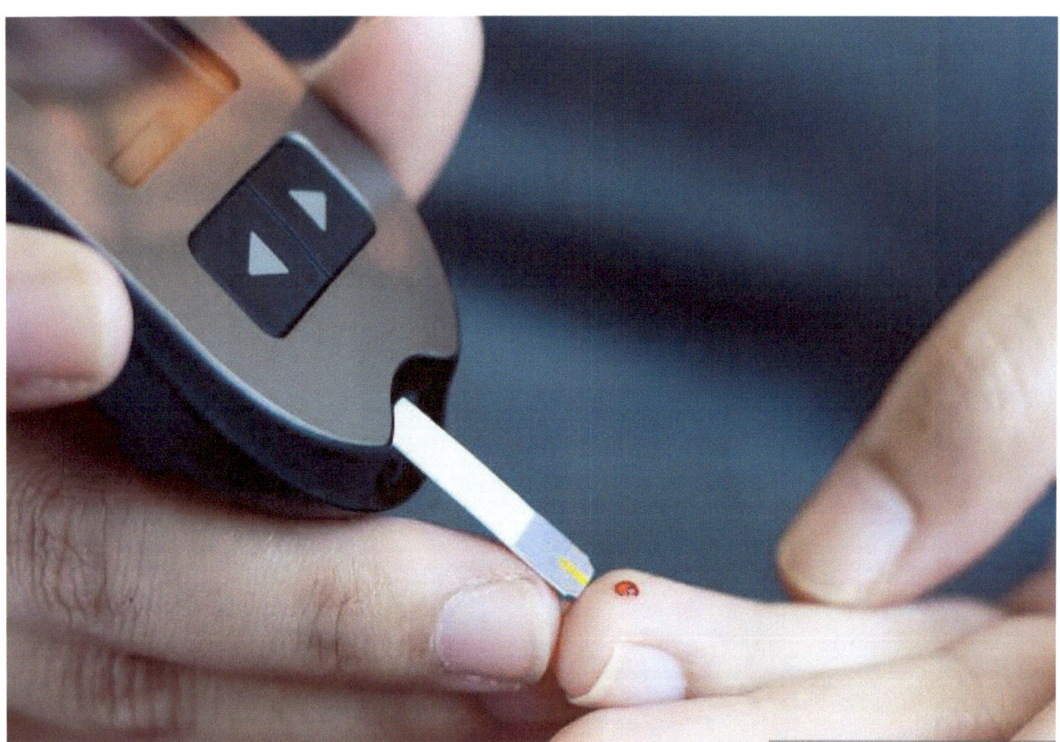

In addition to monitoring your blood sugar levels, it is also important to keep a detailed record of your readings. By keeping a log of your blood sugar levels, along with notes about your diet, exercise, and medication regimen, you can track your progress over time and identify any areas that may need improvement. This information can be invaluable when working with your healthcare team to make adjustments to your treatment plan.

Tracking your blood sugar levels can also help you identify potential triggers that may cause your blood sugar to spike or drop unexpectedly. By pinpointing these triggers, such as certain foods, stressors, or activities, you can take proactive steps to avoid them or make necessary adjustments to prevent blood sugar fluctuations. This level of awareness and control can be empowering and can significantly improve your overall quality of life.

In conclusion, tracking your blood sugar levels is a vital tool in managing and reversing Type 2 diabetes. By monitoring your blood sugar regularly, keeping detailed records, and identifying potential triggers, you can take control of your diabetes and make positive changes to your lifestyle. Remember, knowledge is power when it comes to managing your health, and by staying informed and proactive, you can work towards achieving optimal blood sugar levels and overall wel-being.

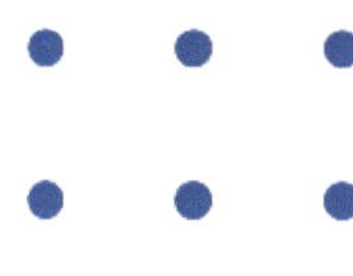

Consulting with Healthcare Providers

Consulting with healthcare providers is a crucial step in the journey of reversing type 2 diabetes. Your healthcare team, consisting of doctors, nurses, dietitians, and other specialists, plays a vital role in guiding you towards better health. When it comes to managing diabetes, it is important to have regular check-ups and consultations with your healthcare providers to monitor your progress and make necessary adjustments to your treatment plan.

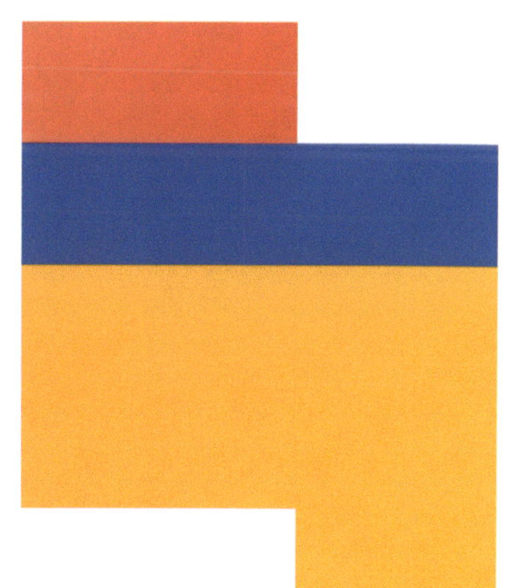

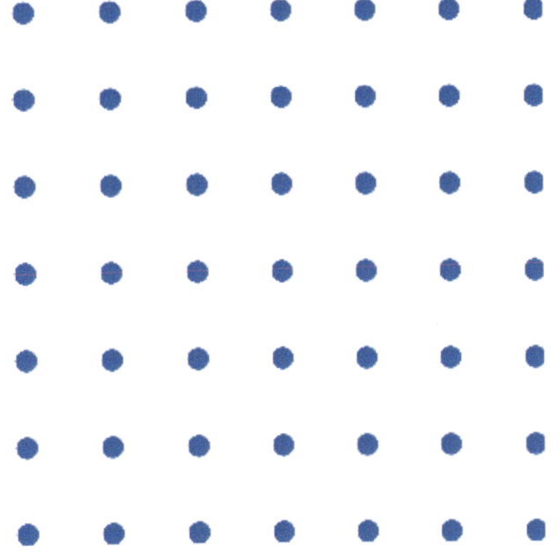

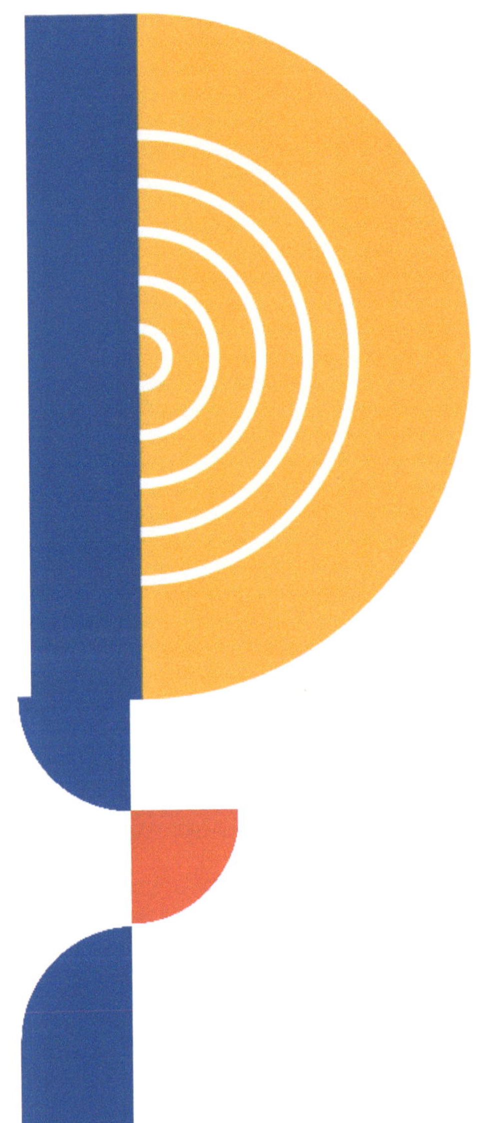

During your consultations, it is important to be open and honest with your healthcare providers about your symptoms, concerns, and goals. They rely on this information to provide you with the best possible care and support. Remember that they are there to help you, so don't hesitate to ask questions or seek clari cation on any aspect of your treatment plan. Your healthcare providers will work with you to develop a personalized treatment plan that suits your individual needs and lifestyle. This plan may include medication, dietary changes, exercise recommendations, and stress management techniques. By following this plan consistently and making necessary lifestyle modi cations, you can improve your blood sugar control and potentially reverse your diabetes.

In addition to medication and other conventional treatments, your healthcare providers may also recommend alternative therapies such as meditation to help manage stress and improve overall wel-being. Meditation has been shown to have numerous health benefits, including reducing blood sugar levels, lowering blood pressure, and promoting relaxation. By incorporating meditation into your daily routine, you can complement your medical treatment and enhance your chances of reversing type 2 diabetes.

Ultimately, consulting with healthcare providers is an essential part of your diabetes reversal journey. By working together with your medical team, staying proactive about your health, and following their recommendations, you can take control of your diabetes and work towards a healthier, happier life. Remember that you are not alone in this journey – your healthcare providers are there to support you every step of the way.

51

Making Sustainable Changes for Long- Term Success

Making sustainable changes for long-term success in type2diabetes reversal is crucial for maintaining a healthy lifestyle. It's not just about making temporary changes to your diet or exercise routine; it's about creating lasting habits that will benefit your health for years to come. By incorporating sustainable changes into your daily routine, you can significantly improve your blood sugar levels and overall well- being. One key sustainable change you can make is to focus on a whole food, plant-based diet. This means consuming plenty of fruits, vegetables, whole grains, and legumes while minimizing processed foods, added sugars, and unhealthy fats. A plant-based diet has been shown to improve insulin sensitivity, lower blood sugar levels, and reduce the risk of developing complications associated with type 2 diabetes. By making this dietary shift, you can create a foundation for long-term success in managing your condition. In addition to changing your diet, incorporating regular physical activity into your routine is essential for long-term success in reversing type 2 diabetes. Exercise helps lower blood sugar levels, improve insulin sensitivity, and promote weight loss, all of which are crucial for managing diabetes effectively. Whether it's walking, swimming, cycling, or yoga, finding an activity you enjoy and can stick with is key to maintaining a sustainable exercise routine.

Another sustainable change you can make is to prioritize stress management and self- care practices in your daily life. Chronic stress can significantly impact blood sugar levels and insulin resistance, making it harder to control diabetes. By incorporating techniques such as meditation, deep breathing, mindfulness, or yoga into your routine, you can reduce stress levels and improve your overall well-being. Prioritizing self-care is essential for long-term success in managing type 2diabetes.

Inconclusion, making sustainable changes for long-term success in reversing type 2 diabetes is crucial for maintaining a healthy lifestyle. By focusing on a **whole food, plant-based diet, regular physical activity, stress management, and self-care practices,** you can significantly improve your blood sugar levels and overall well-being. By incorporating these changes into your daily routine and making them apriority, you can create lasting habits that will benefit your health for years to come.

Chapter 11:
Establishing Road Map for Diabetes Reversal

Road Map for Diabetes Reversal

Reversing diabetes, particularly type 2 diabetes, involves a combination of lifestyle changes, medical interventions, and ongoing monitoring. Here is a structured roadmap to reverse type 2 diabetes from Medication to Meditation:

1. Medical Management:
- **Medical Evaluation:** Comprehensive check-up to confirm diagnosis, understand severity, and identify any complications.
- **Blood Tests:** HbA1c, fasting blood glucose, oral glucose tolerance test (OGTT), lipid profile, and kidney function tests.
- **Treatment:** Some diabetes drugs are more likely to cause Hypoglycemia and Weight gain especially insulin and sulfonylureas. **Metformin, DPP-4 inhibitors, and SGLT2 inhibitors** have a lower risk of Hypoglycemia and Obesity so these are preferred.
- **Medication Review:** Work with a healthcare provider to review current medications and adjust as necessary.
- **Glucose Monitoring:** Regularly monitor blood sugar levels to track progress and make informed decisions.
- **Medication Adherence:** Follow prescribed medication regimens carefully.
- **Healthcare Team:** Regular consultations with doctors, dietitians, diabetes educators, and possibly a mental health professional.
- **Regular Check-Ups:** Frequent follow-ups to monitor progress and make necessary adjustments.

2. Dietary Changes:
- **Balanced Diet:** Emphasize whole foods, such as vegetables, fruits, lean proteins, and whole grains.
- **Low Carbohydrate Diet:** Avoid sugar, refined flour, sugary drinks, white rice, white bread. Monitor and control carbohydrate intake to pr event spikes in blood sugar.
- **Healthy Fats:** Incorporate healthy fats from sources like avocados, nuts, seeds, and olive oil.
- **Lean proteins:** such as poultry, fish, tofu, paneer and legumes should be preferred.
- **High Fiber Diet:** Salads, raw vegetables, millets, fruits are preferred.
- **Portion Control:** Manage portion sizes to avoid overeating.
- **Regular Meals:** Eat at consistent times to help regulate blood sugar levels.
- **Intermittent Fasting:** should be incorporated under supervision of health care professionals.

3. Exercise:
- **Regular Exercise:** Aim for at least 150 minutes of moderate-intensity aerobic exercise per week (e.g., walking, cycling, swimming).
- **Strength Training:** Include resistance exercises at least twice a week.
- **Increase Daily Activity:** Incorporate more physical activity into daily routines (eg.taking stairs, walking instead of driving).

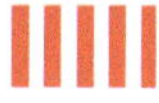

4. **Stress Management:**
   - **Mindfulness and Relaxation:** Practice stress-reduction techniques such as meditation, yoga, or deep breathing exercises.
   - **Mental Health Support:** Seek counselling or therapy if needed to address emotional challenges associated with diabetes management.
   - **Establish a Consistent Sleep Schedule:** by limiting screen time before bedtime, staying active during the day, reducing caffeine intake etc.

5. **Social support for Diabetes patients:**
   - **Support System:** Engage with support groups, family, or friends to stay motivated.

6. **Ongoing Education:**
   - **Stay Informed:** Keep up-to-date with the latest research and recommendations on diabetes management.
   - **Self-Education:** Continue learning about diabetes and how to manage it effectively.

7. **Prevention of Complications**
   Regular Screenings:
   - **Eye Exams:** Annual eye check-ups to monitor for diabetic retinopathy.
   - **Foot Care:** Regular foot exams to prevent and manage complications.
   - **Cardiovascular Health:** Monitor blood pressure and cholesterol levels to reduce the risk of heart disease.

8. **Monitoring Progress:**
   - **Assess Progress:** Regularly evaluate progress towards goals and make adjustments as necessary.
   - **Reflect on Challenges:** Identify and address any obstacles or difficulties encountered.

9. **Celebrate Success**
   - **Milestones:** Celebrate small victories and milestones in your journey towards diabetes reversal.
   - **Positive Reinforcement:** Use positive reinforcement to stay motivated and committed to long-term health.
   Always work closely with healthcare professionals when making significant changes to your health regimen, and ensure that any plan is tailored to your individual needs and circumstances.

References:
1) Standards of care in Diabetes – American Diabetes Association -2023
2) RSSDI Clinical Practice Recommendations for the Management of Type 2 Diabetes Mellitus
3) The Diabetes Code by Dr Jason Fung
4) www.who.int>india>health-topics

Diabetes Reversal: Medication to Meditation

   is a guide that offers a comprehensive approach to managing type 2 diabetes through a combination of medication, nutritional management exercise strategies, yoga and mindfulness practices such as meditation. By taking a holistic approach to your health and well- being, you can empower yourself to take control of your diabetes and potentially reverse its effects. Remember, small changes can lead to big results, so start implementing these key points into your daily routine today for a healthier tomorrow.

Dr Lomeshkumar Thakore
MBBS, PGCIH, CPCDM (RSSDI)

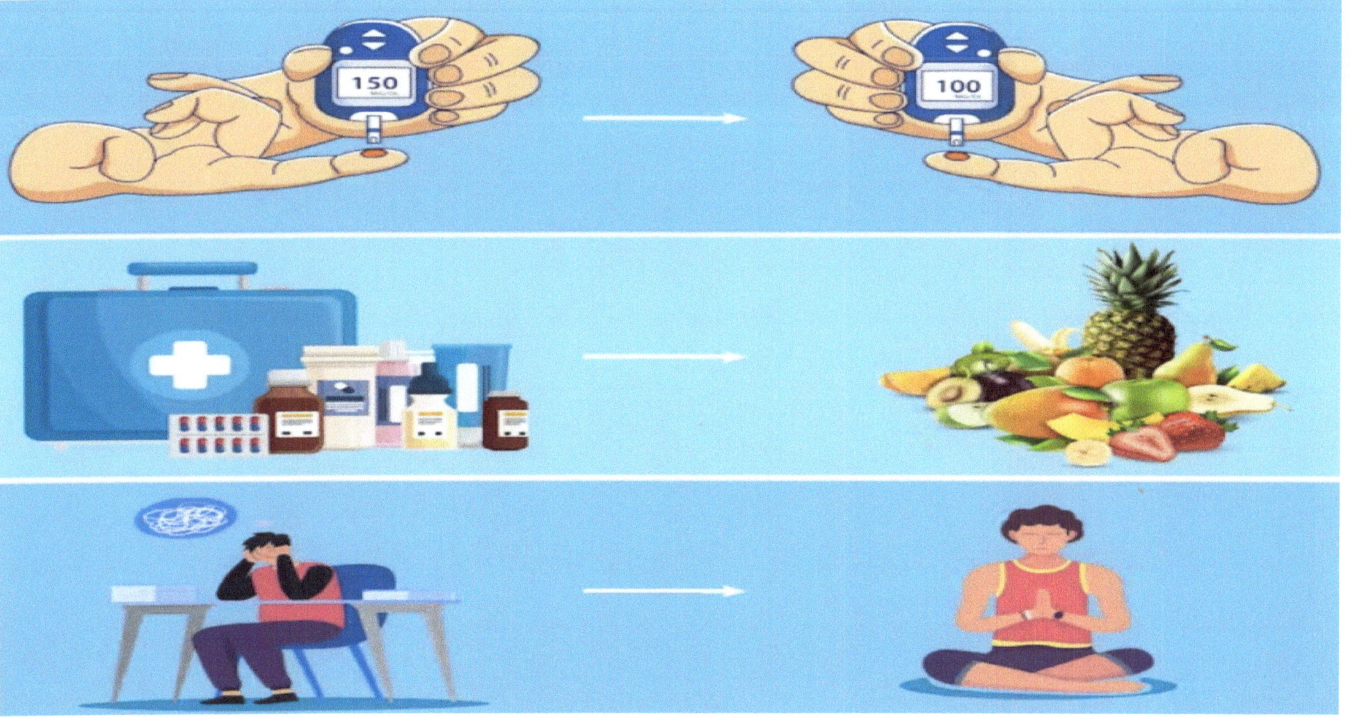

www.ingramcontent.com/pod-product-compliance
Lightning Source LLC
Chambersburg PA
CBHW040047240726
48664CB00004B/1098